BREAST FEEDING

stories to inspire and inform

Published by Lonely Scribe
www.lonelyscribe.co.uk

First published 2012

Cover design and typesetting
copyright © 2012 Armadillo Design Ltd

ISBN: 978-1-905179-04-6

BREAST FEEDING

stories to inspire and inform

Edited by Susan Last

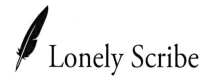

Lonely Scribe

Dedication

To Ray, for everything

Contents

Breastfeeding is an instinctual and natural act, but it is also an art that is learned day by day. The reality is that almost all women can breastfeed, have enough milk for their babies and learn how to overcome problems both large and small. It is almost always simply a matter of practical knowledge and not a question of good luck.

La Leche League

Acknowledgements

I would like to thank everyone who has helped with this project – it has been a real team effort. So thanks to all the contributors who took the time to write up their experiences, or put up with me interviewing them, and thus provided the main part of the text. Thanks also to encouraging friends and publishing/writing colleagues: Tom and Aby Cairns, Lyndsey Miles and Alison Blenkinsop, who checked my introduction for errors. And, of course, thanks to Ray, Evie, Marcus and Ada, for making the book possible in so many ways.

If a multinational company developed a product that was a nutritionally balanced and delicious food, a wonder drug that both prevented and treated disease, cost almost nothing to produce and could be delivered in quantities controlled by the consumers' needs, the very announcement of their find would send their shares rocketing to the top of the stock market. The scientists who developed the product would win prizes and the wealth and influence of everyone involved would increase dramatically. Women have been producing such a miraculous substance, breastmilk, since the beginning of human existence.

Gabrielle Palmer

Introduction

I began work on this collection of breastfeeding stories when my first daughter, Evie, was around six months old. She's now five, has a three-year old brother called Marcus, and I'm breastfeeding their younger sister Ada, who is a year old.

I realised while feeding Evie that the best support I had for breastfeeding (and parenting in general) came from other like-minded people who had 'been there'. I was fortunate to have a very pro-breastfeeding health visitor, but the support of my peers – friends I'd made at NCT classes, a particular friend who was training as a midwife, and a very good friend made at a baby group – was the most critical when things were tough. I realise that, by luck, I had excellent support around me – I'm all too aware that not everyone has the good fortune to have such well-informed and supportive friends and acquaintances. Parenting can seem very lonely when those around you do not understand or appreciate your struggles, and it can be very demoralising to have your firmly-held beliefs swept aside with casual, mis-informed advice: who hasn't heard someone or other say, as if it were the answer to everything 'You could always give him a bottle'?

As time went by the value of peer support for breastfeeding became clearer and clearer to me. When Marcus was breastfeeding I informally supported a couple of mothers who lived near me. My health visitor put me in touch with them and I visited, with Marcus in tow, to chat about breastfeeding. I gave a few tips, and, perhaps most importantly, let them know that what was happening with them and their babies was normal, and that it would get easier. I found it very rewarding, over several weeks, to see people who'd been on the point of giving up breastfeeding really getting to grips with it and overcoming the hurdles they'd been facing.

Shortly after I had Ada I did a course to become a volunteer peer supporter, and for the last year I've been supporting women to breastfeed by taking my turn to answer calls to our helpline, and by attending the baby clinic held in our village. I also run an informal coffee morning for new mums at my house each week. I find supporting other mothers, who are going through many of the struggles I have experienced myself, very satisfying, and the groups and coffee mornings give them chance to create supportive networks of their own. It's great to see them weeks and months down the line, still happily breastfeeding, becoming positive breastfeeding role models for the new mothers that join the groups when their babies are born. All this – rightly – seems a very long way from the unhelpful 'breast v bottle' debates that seem to crop up all the time in the papers and on television. Peer support is not about judging mothers' choices, or breastfeeding evangelism – it's about positive ways of helping those who want to breastfeed, for whom it matters, to continue for as long as they want to, and supporting them to make informed choices for themselves and their families. The central ideas are providing accurate information and offering encouragement, reassurance and support – and these are also the aims of this book.

Over the years it has also become clearer to me how much of a cultural issue breastfeeding is in our society. Reading Gabrielle Palmer's thought-provoking book *The Politics of Breastfeeding* taught me a lot – but it is all around us, and once you become aware of it you can see why we need more effective breastfeeding support in this country. Breastfeeding does not make much in the way of profits for the big baby-feeding companies, and it has virtually no advertising budget. The importance and value of breastfeeding is easily overlooked in a sea of advertising for follow-on milks, first-stage baby foods (badged as suitable from four months despite Department of Health guidelines recommending the introduction of solids from six months), dummies, comforters, baby monitors, expensive pushchairs and all the other paraphernalia new parents are encouraged to believe they need. The increasing availability of breastfeeding accessories: gel-filled breast pads, nursing covers, electric pumps and 'reminder' bracelets, may seem at first glance to be benign, or even useful – but their existence can also be seen to be subtly undermining of breastfeeding's convenience and simplicity, and women's rights to feed their children whenever and wherever they need to. Add into the mix unhelpful media coverage of breastfeeding, our collective angst about feeding in public, the fact that infant feeding is most often characterised by a bottle symbol, and the myths that persist about breastfeeding, and it is not surprising that in our society women can find initiating and maintaining breastfeeding difficult. For much, much more discussion of these issues, please do peruse the further reading lists at the end of the book. It's a fascinating, though at times deeply depressing, issue to explore. My own attempts to bolster a counter-culture of breastfeeding friendliness have been characterised by determined feeding in public to help normalise breastfeeding, by my work as a peer supporter, and, of course, by the production of this book.

Breastfeeding my three children has given me a much deeper understanding of how complex an issue breastfeeding can be. It is not only a physical process, but also an emotional one, for mother and baby, and while it is often both pleasurable and rewarding there are also plenty of potential challenges, which is where good-quality support really comes into its own. One of my main motivations for putting together this book was that I found a gap in the information available to women about breastfeeding. There is plenty of 'how to' material out there. A quick search will turn up endless books that will claim to tell you all you need to know about breastfeeding, with step-by-step diagrams, expert opinions and plenty of sound reasons why you should make the effort.

But what I needed, on my dark days when the baby wouldn't feed well and I wondered whether it was all worth it, was real-life experience. We don't all have mothers, sisters and grandmothers on hand to help us out. We don't all have supportive networks of breastfeeding friends, or understanding health visitors, or concerned partners or husbands. I found great comfort from using online forums, such as Mumsnet, where helpful and experienced mothers could offer a range of solutions to problems I was facing, and in some ways this book is an extension of that idea.

It's naïve to say that breastfeeding is 'easy, cheap, convenient – a no brainer', which is what I thought before I had my first child. Since then I've become very aware of the fact that breastfeeding is, as the La Leche League's famous book on the subject acknowledges, 'a womanly art', with all the variability that implies. There are many ways to achieve 'successful' breastfeeding. Indeed, while compiling this book my own definition of what constitutes successful breastfeeding has changed dramatically. I once thought (uncompromisingly, and before I had children) that successful breastfeeding was defined by the World Health Organisation (WHO) advice: it recommends exclusively breastfeeding to six months, then continuing breastfeeding to two years and beyond. Anything less than this ideal seemed somehow lacking. Time, more children, contact with breastfeeding mothers and personal research has led to me to a completely different, much more sympathetic view. I would argue now that all breastfeeds are valuable – every breastfeed counts, whether it is just one feed of colostrum in the delivery suite, or the last night feed that a walking, talking older child just can't do without. And 'success', for me, is measured by the feelings of the babies and mothers themselves – happy, confident mothers who know that they've made informed decisions that are right for themselves and their families are the best advertisement for breastfeeding, whether they stopped feeding after six weeks, six months or six years. That is not to say that the WHO's advice is wrong, or should be changed: it is an important evidence-based *guideline* that gives valuable health information, and is not a stick with which to beat breastfeeding mothers who for whatever reason did not continue breastfeeding that long.

In this book, more than twenty women tell their own stories of breastfeeding. There is a wide range of experience among them. For some it was an easy, relaxed relationship with the baby from the start, for others it was almost a trial to be endured for the sake of the baby's welfare. Yet all the women have overwhelmingly positive feelings about breastfeeding and are proud of their achievements. In some cases they have overcome extremely complex problems, and have been empowered by their success. Many of the women express surprise at the strength of their own feelings about breastfeeding, or by how much they enjoy breastfeeding – they find something almost primal about it (which is logical, when you think about it, as breastfeeding is the normal behaviour of our species).

It is very clear from the stories that the differences between babies, and people's situations, are enormous – and our expectations of breastfeeding are often badly skewed. Rather than thinking of breastfeeding as something with concrete answers, or dos and don'ts, it can be more helpful to think of the existence of a range of normal breastfeeding behaviours, with each mum and baby pair ending up somewhere on the spectrum. For example, you may breastfeed exclusively and have a baby who sleeps for seven hours at night and is sick after every feed, while your neighbour may breastfeed exclusively and have a baby who wakes every two hours to feed and poos every seven days or so. Your experiences are very different, but in both cases the breastfeeding is working fine, even if the patterns of behaviour might not seem ideal to the mothers.

Wherever you fit in along the spectrum of breastfeeding experience, there are bound to be feelings and situations in this book that will strike a chord. My hope is that these women's stories about the realities of breastfeeding their babies will help others to see how it could work, or continue to work, for them. I'm also very aware that sometimes, for mothers who are struggling, it's just one person, saying one thing at just the right time, that can make all the difference, and I hope that mothers in need of a word of encouragement may find what they need in these pages.

As for inspiration – for the subtitle of the book is 'stories to inspire and inform' – I encourage you to look out for the many beautiful moments described by mothers in their stories. Whether it's the incredible feeling of closeness during night feeds with a tiny, snuggly newborn, or the immense feeling of pride (mixed with a little sadness) when an older child finally stops breastfeeding, there are such genuine emotions expressed here that they can't help but touch others.

Exploding some common myths

It can be very difficult to sort out fact from fiction with regard to breastfeeding. Advice comes from many quarters: health professionals (midwives, health visitors, doctors, paediatricians), other mothers (the older generation and your contemporaries), breastfeeding support workers (helplines, support groups) parenting literature (magazines and books) and just about everyone else too. It is a subject on which everyone seems to have an opinion, and proper, evidence-based information can be hard to come by. Different advisors give conflicting information and this is certainly apparent in the stories that follow.

Obviously each mother needs to make her own decisions – but how is she to get access to the information she needs if those advising her do not agree? Here are some brief points to bear in mind – but for more detailed information do see the suggestions for further reading at the end of the book.

Training

This is especially relevant in the context of health professionals. Midwives generally do have some training in breastfeeding, particularly if the hospital has 'baby friendly' status. Maternity assistants, health visitors and even doctors and paediatricians, as unbelievable as it sounds, may not have any formal training in breastfeeding, or supporting breastfeeding, and what knowledge they do have may be outdated or just plain wrong. It is worth bearing this in mind if you are having problems. If in doubt, ask to be referred to someone who does have the knowledge you need. This might be a midwife who has received additional training, an infant feeding advisor based at the hospital, or a breastfeeding counsellor from one of the breastfeeding charities (contact details for these can be found at the end of the book).

Outdated advice

Other mothers, including your own mother and your contemporaries, can make or break your breastfeeding experience. Support and encouragement from them can be invaluable, but you may also be given outdated or wrong information. Comments such as 'Have you got her onto four-hourly feeds yet?' 'That baby is hungry, you're always feeding him' and 'Why don't you let me have her for a few hours so you can get a sleep?' may be made with good intentions, but nonetheless undermine breastfeeding because they are based on outdated ideas. Newborn babies need frequent access to the breast for food and comfort to help get breastfeeding well established, and babies are less stressed and feed better if the mother responds quickly to feeding cues (looking around for mum, sucking hands, smacking lips) before crying starts. New mothers should be supported in other ways to ensure they get enough rest – if family members can take over household chores, care of other children and preparation of meals for a while, mum and baby can take it easy.

The normal course of breastfeeding

Because our culture is not supportive of breastfeeding, and bottle-feeding is commonplace, many women have no idea of what constitutes 'normal' breastfeeding and do not know what to expect from it in the first few days and weeks, or later on. They compare breastfed infants to their bottle-fed peers and assume they must be doing something wrong, when in fact all is well. The first few weeks, while breastfeeding is established, can be challenging. The baby may feed very frequently, may wake often for feeds at night, and may 'cluster feed' – pinning you to the sofa for what seems like hours – in the early evening. But if you can get through these first few weeks, then the months ahead can be truly satisfying – relaxed, easy breastfeeding, no need for bottles or other equipment, no expense of formula milk. Routines, spacing of feeds, dummies, bottles and teats can all interfere with the normal course of breastfeeding and should be treated with caution. Breastfeeding is a supply and demand system: if you miss out feeds (by delaying them, or replacing with formula and not pumping) your body will respond by making less milk. Babies may get used to the faster flow and feel of the bottle teat and then be fussy or appear to reject the breast as it is so different (whatever the bottle and teat advertisers may say!). These things can lead to reduced milk supply and an early end to breastfeeding – something it is important to be aware of if continuing to breastfeed is important to you.

It seems to be a pervasive view in our society that bottle-fed babies sleep for longer than those who are breastfed, and it is a common reason for mothers to switch to formula, often beginning with a bottle at bedtime (see worries about supply, below) in the hope that the baby will 'go a bit longer'. In fact the best research that we currently have suggests that breastfeeding mothers get more sleep than bottle-feeding mothers – partly because of the hormones released when feeding that enable both you and your baby to fall asleep more quickly afterwards, and partly because of the reduced amount of time spent on the feeding. Research also shows that night feeds are important for maintaining your milk supply in the longer term (hence the advice given to mothers who are pumping to ensure that they pump during the night). Rather than blaming breastfeeding for our wakeful babies, it would be more helpful for mothers if we were honest about the fact that different babies have different sleep habits, so expecting them all to sleep through the night without feedings from six months, or nine months, or a year can just be one more source of anxiety for mothers. Sometimes it is easier to modify your own expectations (and sleeping arrangements!) than to change your baby's habits. For much more on this, and breastfeeding-friendly sleep advice, see Elizabeth Pantley's *The No-Cry Sleep Solution*.

The fact that breastfeeding is both food and comfort for babies – and not just newborns but older babies and toddlers too – can sometimes cause mothers to worry that they are somehow instilling 'bad habits' in their babies by feeding them until they fall asleep, either for naps or at bedtime, or feeding them when they are upset, or cold, or have had a fright, or just for closeness. Outdated ideas (see above) are often responsible for these worries. We now know that babies with secure attachments, whose needs (for food and comfort) are readily met, are more likely to grow up happy and confident. And for busy mothers, breastfeeding for comfort can be the most useful tool in the box – if a company marketed a product that could soothe babies to sleep, calm their crying, fill their tummies and help ensure their future mental health, it would be flying off the shelves. Breastfeeding mothers have no need for such a product: they have it readily available, at the right temperature and the right price (free!).

As babies get older and better at breastfeeding you may notice feeds becoming shorter – don't panic that they are not getting enough milk! As babies grow they feed more efficiently and some can take all they want in only a few minutes. Many people worry about supply in the evenings, when breasts seem soft, but that too is normal – evening milk is higher in fat and lower in volume than daytime milk. Breasts are never 'empty' – milk production is a continuous process – and the more you feed, the more milk your body will produce. It can be hard to have confidence in a process you can't see, so if you need encouragement talk to other breastfeeding mothers or supporters before worrying too much.

Another source of worry is the foremilk/hindmilk question – it's something that is often poorly understood and mothers are left worrying that their babies are not getting all the 'full fat' milk that they need, perhaps because the baby does not seem to be on the breast for very long (see the point above about older babies feeding more quickly). There is no exact point in a feeding (after a certain number of minutes, for example) when the milk changes from foremilk (thirst-quenching) to hindmilk (richer and fattier) – rather it happens gradually, with the fat content of the milk increasing as the feed goes on. Generally, if you 'finish the first breast first', letting the baby suckle for as long as he or she likes, before offering the second breast, then you never have to worry about foremilk and hindmilk. If the baby takes only a very small amount from the second breast, start the next feeding on that side. Some babies take only one side at each feed, some take both, some finish the second and want to go back on the first again! Again, if you are worried ask for reassurance from someone experienced.

Weaning is an area of great concern for mothers – there is so much 'advice' that it can become very confusing. Bear in mind that magazines would not exist without advertisers who want to sell baby food and accessories – this has an impact on the editorial content. The Department of Health guidelines, as most people know, are to breastfeed exclusively for the first six months, and then to add appropriate solid foods. As mentioned earlier, this is a guideline, not an absolute rule – but it does give valuable health information. We know that if babies are given solid food too early it can put them at risk of health problems later on. If breastmilk is replaced with puréed fruit and vegetables too early, the baby can actually be at a nutritional disadvantage – breastmilk is higher in calories and essential nutrients than these common first foods. The best information we now have suggests that most babies will be ready for solid foods at around six months. The signs that a baby is ready are that they have lost their tongue-thrust reflex (which will push food out of the mouth), that they can sit up, perhaps with a little support but with good head control, in a highchair or on a lap, and that they can reach out and grasp food and bring it to their mouths. Taking more milk feeds, waking up in the night when they have previously slept through and chewing on fists or mouthing objects are not signs that a baby is ready for solid foods, although they are often taken as such.

A baby starting solids at around six months, who is breastfeeding well, needs no complex weaning regime – you can simply start to offer foods from your plate, at times when you will be eating. They will let you know, by reaching out and grabbing, what they want to try! At around six months much of the outdated advice about weaning: start with fruit and vegetable purées, add baby rice to milk, then gradually introduce textured food, does not apply at all. Your baby can have meat and fish, pasta, potatoes, fruits and vegetables, fingers of toast, hard-boiled egg – almost anything you would eat can be adapted by leaving out added salt and sugar. And they can feed themselves – there is no need for 'here comes the spoon' type performances. Many mothers worry about how much their children are eating – if they are breastfeeding well then it doesn't really matter how much they eat at first – they will still be getting nearly all of their nutrition from breastmilk. As they eat increasing amounts of food (you'll be able to tell by the poo!) they will gradually reduce the amount of breastmilk they take, although you may not notice this for some time. This approach to weaning is known as 'baby-led' weaning and is the ideal way to follow on from breastfeeding. For much more on the subject see the resources at the end of the book, in particular Gill Rapley and Tracey Murkett's excellent book *Baby-Led Weaning – Helping Your Baby To Love Good Food.*

Your diet and health while breastfeeding

To scotch a few common misconceptions: breastmilk is rarely if ever unsafe, whatever the mother may have been eating. Formula milk carries many more risks. With most diets, apart from true starvation (as shown by research into malnourished refugee mothers and their babies), breastmilk quality and quantity is unaffected. Your body will use some of its stores of nutrients to nourish the baby. However, a healthy balanced diet, with minimal alcohol, will certainly help give you the energy and alertness you need to care for your baby. From the point of view of your baby's health, it would be ideal to consider a diet low in toxins well before conception, and continuing throughout pregnancy and breastfeeding (this is why pregnant women are advised not to eat shark, swordfish and marlin!).

Smokers should still breastfeed. In fact, for babies of committed smokers breastfeeding is even more important to help counteract some of the risks of passive smoking (eg SIDS), and smokers can reduce the risks further by timing their cigarette breaks and avoiding bed-sharing. (See the Breastfeeding Network – contact details at the end of the book – for more information.)

Most medical conditions can be treated with drugs that are compatible with breastfeeding, although many doctors are unable or unwilling to do the necessary research – contact the Breast-feeding Network pharmacy advice line for help. It is possible to breastfeed while receiving treatment for many illnesses and con-ditions, and also to continue to breastfeed despite surgery (for you or the baby). For much more information on these topics, see the list of further reading, in particular chapters in Dr Jack Newman's *Ultimate Breastfeeding Book of Answers*. I would suggest that whenever anyone suggests that you should give up breast-feeding, that you push them further to explain why, and seek further advice/opinions before taking them seriously.

A note on the breastfeeding stories

The stories that appear here are 'straight from the horse's mouth': they have not been substantially edited. This has caused me one problem: at times mothers report advice they have been given, from friends or health professionals, or state as facts things that they personally believe about breastfeeding, which are inconsistent with the best evidence-based knowledge currently available. What is an editor to do in such a situation? I wanted to allow women to speak for themselves, and to baldly correct their beliefs, or to rubbish advice that might, even if misdirected, have contributed to them continuing to breastfeed, seemed to deny the reality of their experiences. And yet it does readers no favours to perpetuate potentially unhelpful myths. What I have done, in order to flag up to readers where such inconsistencies occur, is to mark problematic text with an asterisk, which indicates that the matter in question is discussed in the 'Exploding some common myths' section. The books, websites and helplines mentioned at the end of the book are all reliable sources of information about breastfeeding for readers who want to do further research themselves.

When we trust the makers of baby formula more than we do our own ability to nourish our babies, we lose a chance to claim an aspect of our power as women. Thinking that baby formula is as good as breast milk is believing that thirty years of technology is superior to three million years of nature's evolution. Countless women have regained trust in their bodies through nursing their children, even if they weren't sure at first that they could do it. It is an act of female power, and I think of it as feminism in its purest form.

Christine Northrup

Susan's story

When the midwife asked me, at my booking-in appointment, whether I intended to breastfeed, I said yes immediately. It had always seemed a no-brainer to me: best for baby, best for mum, easy, cheap, natural, environmentally friendly. In retrospect I had no idea whatsoever about what to expect – my knowledge of breastfeeding, like most first-time mums, was completely hazy. I knew that my mother had breastfed me (against the odds, in 1970s America!) and that my grandmothers, with eight children between them, had breastfed all their children.

Evie was born in July 2006 and I was lucky enough to have a fabulous home birth with a short and relatively painless labour – she arrived within six hours of the first contraction in a birth pool on our landing, with no pain relief, no stitches and no complications. So far so good. She was put to the breast straight away, but she was pretty sleepy and although she eventually latched on for a few sucks, she did not feed very well on that first day.

I soon realised that it wasn't just the baby who needed to learn how to breastfeed, it was me as well. I found it hard to find a position that felt natural for holding her to the breast, even with pillows, and at first I could only ever get her to latch on to one side. For several days, each time the midwife or the maternity assistant came to see us, I would have to ask again for help with latching Evie on.

When my milk came in on the third day my breasts became enormous – before pregnancy I was a 32B and that day I think I was giving Jordan a run for her money! My breasts were rock solid and hot with the milk and Evie was still sleepy and reluctant to feed well. In retrospect a breast pump would have helped me to feel more comfortable, but at the time I was very reluctant to introduce anything 'unnatural', because I'd read so much about the importance of getting feeding properly established, so I stuck to expressing tiny amounts by hand and putting hot flannels on my breasts to encourage them to leak.

Right from the beginning Evie preferred the left breast to the right, which is apparently very common, and as the days went by I was worried that she might never feed properly from the right-hand side. However, as we got more used to each other she did feed better from that side, although she always preferred the left.

In the early days feeding was a messy business – milk got everywhere. It would leak from my breasts all the time anyway, but when Evie fed she would often suck for a short while, then let go, and milk would spray out of the nipple all over me and across her face. I couldn't feed her without having at least one muslin and a drink of water nearby, but when she cried I would often sit down hurriedly without either of these essential items.

By the time Evie was five weeks old it was clear that she was not a happy and contented baby, and it seemed to be connected to feeding. She would cry and seem uncomfortable after feeds despite our best efforts to wind her. The doctor and health visitor thought it was colic and we embarked on a saga of trying different colic remedies with little to no success. The best thing we could do was to put Evie in the sling – she would sleep well in there and it seemed to ease her discomfort.

I carried on trying to feed Evie as best I could and read all sorts of books and articles. I learned a lot about breastfeeding, but not a lot that helped us. As time went by Evie became even more distressed when feeding. She would feed alright when she was drowsy, but during the day she would often pop off frequently during feeds, and she would arch her back and cry in pain. At times she and I were both in tears by the end of a feed and I worried constantly that she wasn't getting enough milk. She was slow to get over the slight jaundice that she'd had since birth, and she put weight on slowly. She had plenty of wet and dirty nappies, and didn't seem dehydrated, but she didn't seem to be really thriving either. I was frequently at the doctors with her when she refused feeds or seemed particularly uncomfortable, but nothing was seriously enough wrong to really ring any alarm bells.

Over the next few months breastfeeding was really challenging and I felt very disheartened about it. I desperately wanted to feed Evie successfully because I knew how important it was for her health, and it was central to how I thought about myself as a mother. She was difficult to feed in public, what with the popping on and off and the milk spraying everywhere, and she cried a lot during feeds. That really upset me because I always thought of feeding as a comforting experience for a baby. Evie never fell

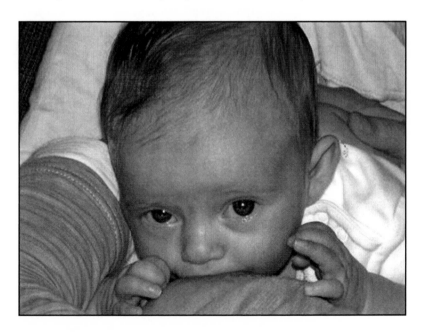

asleep while feeding, and often stayed awake for up to an hour after a feed, even in the middle of the night, because she was too uncomfortable to sleep.

I think the only reason I didn't give up breastfeeding was because I couldn't see how giving up could do her any good. There was no reason to think that formula or bottles would improve her digestive problems. She wouldn't drink from a bottle at all anyway, even for expressed milk. Nor would giving up have done me any good. Although I was worn out and unhappy about our feeding experience, I would have felt as if I'd really failed if I'd given up.

Once, when I actually had Evie latched on and feeding well, sitting up in bed in the middle of the night, I suddenly felt the tickle of spider's legs on my upper arm, on the side I was feeding Evie. I couldn't move – I desperately wanted not to disturb her peaceful feeding, which was so rare, but I couldn't bear the thought of the spider on me, having a lifelong phobia of them. I reached across to my right upper arm with my left hand and brushed firmly downwards, dislodging the spider. I never saw it, but I heard it hit the ground – it must have been a big one. I shuddered, but was glad I had kept Evie latched on throughout!

I tried everything I could to improve Evie's feeding. I would feed her bouncing on the gym ball that I'd had for pregnancy and labour, and that would sometimes help. Or I would walk around while feeding. I would give her a dummy to calm her, then whip it out and stick the nipple in instead – sometimes that worked. I tried feeding naked, feeding lying down, feeding in the 'football' hold, feeding in a darkened room. I tried expressing some milk to dampen the let-down. Nothing really made a difference but each new thing I tried kept me going a bit longer.

Most alarming were the total nursing strikes. Evie would have days when she would barely feed at all, screaming and arching her back whenever I put her to the breast, and I would feel as if I'd spent the entire day trying to get her to suckle. Several times I ended up at the doctors with her and a couple of times she fed well in the surgery as if to prove me wrong.

In the midst of all the feeding difficulties I was immensely grateful for the support of the friends I'd made at NCT classes. All eight of the women in our group successfully breastfed their babies, and all of us were still feeding at six months. In the early days we used to meet for coffee each week at someone's house and that was lovely, sitting there feeding and talking about what was going on with the babies. Quite early on we hit on the idea of going out for lunch at a local pub, which was large, light and airy and where we could get a table with space around it for the babies to sit asleep in their car-seats, although there were always two or three awake and feeding while we ate our lunch, even in the very early days. Later the babies would sit in high chairs or on laps. I don't think any of us had any problems feeding in public and it must have been partly down to the confidence we got from our shared outings. One weekend, when the babies were a couple of months old, we all walked about five miles along the Tissington Trail in the Peak District with our buggies, slings and back carriers. At the tea kiosk above Ashbourne all the girls sat down and latched on the babies – anyone passing must have thought they were at some sort of breastfeeding convention! These meetings tailed off a bit when we started going back to work once the babies were a bit older, but I think we all found them invaluable at the time.

Evie's weight gain continued to be poor and eventually (thank goodness) we were referred to a paediatrician. Ray and I felt as if it was our last chance to help Evie with her feeding problems and we even resorted to videoing a feed to show the consult-ant. By this time Evie was nearly five months old and I knew he would suggest weaning her. I was reluctant to start weaning before six months, having taken on board the advice, but by our second appointment with the consultant, at which he also prescribed infant Gaviscon, I was ready to try anything to help her. So at Christmas, when Evie was exactly five months old, we started her on solid foods, beginning with things like mashed potato and other puréed root vegetables and fruits. She took to the new foods brilliantly, and with the combination of the Gaviscon and the solid food the breastfeeding finally began to improve.

As she had increasing amounts of solid food, Evie gradually began to take fewer breastfeeds. Since she'd never been a very happy feeder, she wasn't reluctant to let the feeds go and I was soon down from six or seven feeds a day to just four: early morning, mid-morning, mid-afternoon and bedtime. However, thanks to the Gaviscon these feeds were trouble-free and I began to really enjoy breastfeeding in a way I'd almost thought I never would. I joked with friends who were giving up after six months that I was carrying on for another six, because the first six months had been so rubbish!

Because I was enjoying feeding so much it was a disappointment to me when, at around eight and a half months, Evie started dropping more breastfeeds. It's strange – it was both heartening, because I knew I was feeding her a good diet and that she was eating well, but upsetting because she was showing signs of self-weaning when I would happily have gone on feeding her for well over a year. At this time she also went through a mercifully brief phase of biting my nipple – her teeth were new and she was keen to try them out. I used to take her off the breast immediately and put her down for a minute or two before trying again, but I couldn't bring myself to be too forceful about ending feeds because I didn't want to put her off.

At ten months Evie started refusing her feed before bed. She'd just whimper when I offered her the breast. I felt a bit unhappy about this seeming 'rejection', and I worried about how I would settle her to sleep at night, but my fears were groundless. Instead of a feed, Evie had a cuddle and a lullaby and went off to sleep fairly reliably. She carried on with a quick feed first thing in the morning for another three weeks before refusing that as well.

So at one week shy of eleven months Evie self-weaned. I know I could have tried to continue with breastfeeding for longer, but I would have felt as if I was trying to get her to do it against her will. I miss feeding her now its finished but I do feel much happier about breastfeeding coming to an end than I would have done if we'd have stopped much earlier on when things were tough. I wish I'd known earlier that it was reflux causing her problems, but in the end she still had the best start because I persevered with the breastfeeding despite all the problems.

*****

When Marcus was born in April 2008, I felt very confident about breastfeeding. All the problems I'd had feeding Evie had meant that I'd done so much research that I felt very well-informed, and I was sure that if I did have problems I would be able to resolve them, either on my own or by contacting the breastfeeding helplines for advice.

I was lucky enough to have another straightforward birth, again at home, and Marcus had his first feed at under an hour old, on the sofa in our living room. He latched on straight away and had a good strong suck, and he seemed much less sleepy than his sister had been. At nearly 8lbs he was a lot bigger than Evie had been and he seemed robust and hungry right from the start. I had been hand expressing colostrum from a few weeks before the birth to help get things moving, and I was hoping to avoid the painful engorgement I'd had when my milk came in the first time. I also had a breast pump at the ready if necessary!

Marcus was born at home on a Saturday morning, and he slept fine (waking three times for a feed) on Saturday night, but by Sunday night he was beside himself, crying constantly despite my putting him to the breast whenever he cried. He was up all night, crying inconsolably, and we rapidly exhausted our (we thought) comprehensive repertoire of tactics to settle him. Eventually we started to get worried, as we'd tried everything we could think of, and having been born at home he had not yet been checked over by a doctor. It genuinely didn't occur to us that he might be hungry and frustrated with only colostrum, but that was what our GP thought when we took him to see her first thing on the Monday morning.

Reassured we took him home. My milk came in later that night and from then on I just fed Marcus whenever and wherever possible. It soon felt like second nature again. I'd worried about what I would do trying to feed Marcus with my toddler running around and demanding my attention, but having baby-proofed the living room and installed a baby-gate across the door, I would park us all in there while I fed him, and distract Evie with books, television or toys as much as I could. She used to like to stroke Marcus's head while he was feeding, which was sweet, but used to put him off! Fortunately Marcus was a very efficient feeder, normally having finished both sides within ten or fifteen minutes, so it never felt like I was pinned to the sofa in quite the same way as I had been when Evie was a newborn.

Evie had been in nursery before Marcus was born, after I'd gone back to work, and we managed to keep her there during my maternity leave. This was great because it kept things 'normal' for her, and gave her some space without Marcus, and I had some days with Marcus where I could just be with him, feed him

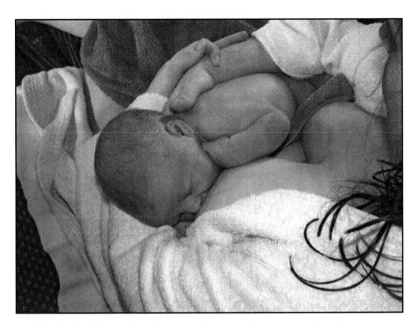

unhurriedly, and take him to friends' houses and baby groups just as I had with Evie while I was on leave with her. I was fortunate to have one very good friend who'd had her second baby just three weeks before Marcus arrived, and we enjoyed our maternity leave together, pushing buggies round the park, then feeding the babies in public in the café while waiting for our jacket potatoes and tea to arrive. I think the café owners might have begun to think of us as 'those mad breastfeeding women' and, once the babies were older and we started baby-led weaning, their hearts probably sank when we walked in, knowing the mess we would leave around the highchairs.

When Marcus was about sixteen weeks old I had a call from my very pro-breastfeeding health visitor. She'd tried her best to help me with Evie's problems, and was really glad that feeding Marcus was going so smoothly. She said she had a mum on her books, in my village, who was struggling with breastfeeding although there was nothing clinically wrong, and she wondered whether I would get in touch with her to offer some support. When Evie was born she'd put me in touch with another mum in the village, and we're still friends now, so I knew the value of getting to know other mums in the early days. I gave the mum a call and asked her what was going on with the feeding. She was experiencing feelings I recognised all too well – she was tired, breastfeeding wasn't easy, she wasn't enjoying it, she was worried the baby wasn't getting enough milk. I went round to see her and her husband, taking Marcus with me, and ended up not only trying to offer some supportive advice, but also giving a practical demonstration. In the next few weeks I saw her a few times, and she came round to see me, and she really got to grips with the breastfeeding, which was great to see. It made me realise (even more) just how valuable peer support can be. I was really glad when the health visitor put me in touch with another mum whom I could help.

Marcus carried on feeding enthusiastically and I started baby-led weaning when he was about twenty-four weeks old, after he literally grabbed a banana out of my hand and mashed it into his face. He still fed several times during the day, and during the night as well, but at that stage I wasn't unduly concerned about the nights, although I would have loved more sleep! My husband and I found ways to cope with it, with him sleeping in another room and looking after Evie, who seldom woke at night, and me looking after Marcus, who still slept in a cot in our room. In the early morning, after a very broken night, I would hand Marcus over to Ray and grab another hour's sleep, which would be enough to keep me going. As he got older we hoped he would sleep more, but the warmth and comfort of milk in the night was just too much for him to give up, and, although I was tired, I still loved the night feeds, in a way. It's a very special feeling to pick up a warm, sleepy baby, feed them blissfully back to sleep and then ease them back peacefully into bed. We moved house when Marcus was just over a year old, which perhaps delayed us doing anything about his night-time sleeping. Eventually, when he was nearly sixteen months old, we decided we couldn't live with the sleep deprivation any longer – it was time to night-wean. In the end it was surprisingly straightforward: Ray looked after Marcus at night for five nights straight, and there was no feeding after the last feed at bedtime. This seemed to do the job and he was soon sleeping longer stretches.We debated whether to try giving up breastfeeding altogether, but I didn't feel ready for that as Marcus still seemed to love it so much. So I carried on doing a last feed before bed. This continued until Marcus was about eighteen months old, when for some reason I wasn't around at bedtime and he went to bed when Ray put him down without a murmur. He never asked to feed again after that, even when I was on bedtime duty.

I found feeding Marcus for so long to be rewarding. It was nice to discover, by virtue of going to a wedding when he was fourteen months old, leaving him in the care of his grandparents, that he would settle for the night, and indeed survive the night, without breastfeeding. He went to nursery three days a week when he was a year old, as Evie had, with no problems and no formula – they simply offered him cows' milk or water when he was there, and I fed him when he was with me. He was definitely able, even at that age, to realise that breastfeeds only happened with me, and to be content with alternatives when I wasn't available. It probably also helped that he was a good eater of solids, but I've come to the conclusion that extended breastfeeding can be a lot more flexible than many believe. Certainly feeding Marcus at eighteen months (one feed before bed, perhaps one feed in the day if he was poorly, or especially upset) was nothing like feeding a newborn, or a six-month-old, or even a year-old baby. I never felt at all odd about feeding my walking, (almost) talking toddler – I think when you've been feeding them all along it just evolves and doesn't seem strange.

When Marcus eventually gave up his bedtime feed I was, as I had been with Evie, a little sad that breastfeeding was over, but at the same time glad that the transition had been made without real upset on either side.

*****

When I was pregnant with my third child I looked forward to a new breastfeeding experience. Both my children were excited about the new arrival and fascinated by the idea that I would be breastfeeding again. Evie asked a lot of questions about how the milk gets into my breasts!

My third baby, Ada, was again born at home in water after a quick labour. She latched on straight away, while I was lying back on a bed propped up with pillows, holding her in skin-to skin. I now know that this is known as 'biological nurturing' and the ideal way to get mothers and babies off to a good start – the skin contact between mother and baby unlocks instinctive behaviour in both of them that leads to babies latching on well. Ada in fact both weed and pooed meconium all over me while I was feeding her – it was quickly wiped away, but perhaps a sign that she'd got a good mouthful of colostrum!

With Ada I felt like I really did know what I was doing and I had been looking forward to getting breastfeeding established again. I hadn't really envisaged any problems at all so I was slightly surprised to find myself dealing with problem engorgement and sore nipples in the first couple of weeks. The two were linked, I think – engorged breasts make it harder for the baby to get a good latch, leading to soreness. I think the engorgement is down to a problem I have with oversupply and fast letdown

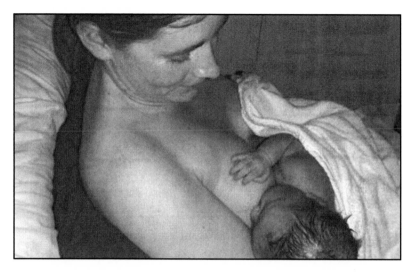

– which seems to get worse with each baby! I worked hard on getting the latch right, and tried all the tricks I'd learned with Evie to work on the engorgement. One new thing that worked well for me was 'reverse pressure softening' – look it up for more information! – which involves pressing back the areola towards the chest with the fingers to encourage the nipple to protrude and enable the baby to latch. I did enough to make it possible for Ada to feed, but nonetheless struggled with the engorgement for a good week or two. Just when I was starting to wonder whether she had a tongue-tie, the situation improved as my supply settled down enough to sort out the engorgement.

In the first few weeks feeds with Ada were messy and not very discreet – the oversupply and fast letdown means that the milk spurts out all over the place, and Ada would often let go just at the moment that the milk let down and cause me to have to hastily mop up with the muslin and try to avoid squirting the person sitting next to me! I knew this would resolve itself as she got older and more able to cope with the fast flow, and by nineteen weeks it was no longer a problem.

With three young children in the house and a lot of lifestyle changes (Evie started school when Ada was eight weeks old, and Marcus started a new pre-school at the same time), I found the ease and convenience of breastfeeding more important than ever. The upside of fast letdown is quick feeds, and I found that if I just topped Ada up before I needed to go anywhere she would be content and sleep in the buggy as I got used to dashing back and forwards to school and pre-school.

Of all my children Ada was the most contented sleeper as a newborn – she woke only once or twice at night from birth until about three months, and slept well during the day on all her outings to fetch and carry the other children. At about three and a half months she started waking much more frequently at night, and I was grateful to be able to soothe her back to sleep by breastfeeding. She was scratching her head and waking herself up, and she was eventually diagnosed with eczema. Treating that

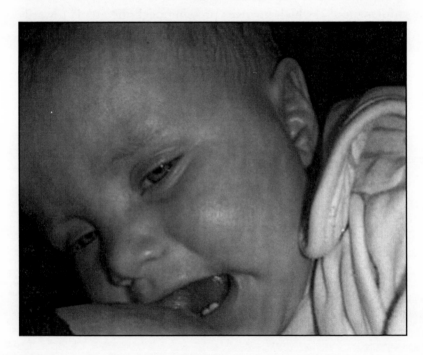

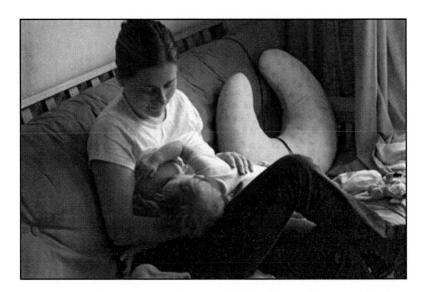

improved her sleep again for a while. Just like when I had Marcus we arranged the household to accommodate the baby, with Ray sleeping in the spare room and looking after Evie and Marcus at night, giving me the flexibility to co-sleep with Ada if she was hard to settle. She mostly slept in bed with me until she was four months old and we started a vague night-time routine with her (her eczema meant she needed a bath and creams applied each night, after which she'd feed to sleep and stay settled for two or three hours), when we started putting her down in her cot.

When Ada was only six weeks old I asked my new health visitor (we had moved house since Marcus was born) whether there were any breastfeeding groups or 'buddy' schemes in our local area, as I was keen to help other mothers if I could. It turned out that a training course for peer supporters was starting just two weeks later, at a local Children's Centre, with a crèche for older children. I wasn't sure I'd be able to fit it in, with all the changes at home and an eight-week old baby, but equally I thought I'd regret it if I didn't. The training was fascinating and I'm now 'qualified' to offer peer support and have begun helping mums in my local area, which is a great feeling. Apart from the satisfaction of helping mums feed the way they want to, it feels to me as if I am doing something practical that is consistent with my view that, in general, the more breastfeeding that goes on, the better.

Ada is now eighteen months old and I'm still breastfeeding – she's just started going to nursery two days a week, and seems to be coping without milk in the day while she's away from me. She still wakes for feeds in the night, and co-sleeps the later part of the night with me. It seems strange to think that I might be approaching the end of breastfeeding when it has been so central to our family life over the last few years. There's no doubt I will look back at it as one of my most precious experiences of motherhood.

Eleanor's story

Whilst I was pregnant, I didn't really consider any possibility other than breastfeeding my baby, having read that breastfeeding would provide massive health benefits for my child. So when I heard at my NCT antenatal class that breastfeeding can be scuppered by various events in the days after birth, I felt quite anxious. I went into the birth worried that the midwife might put my baby off breastfeeding by forcing her face into my breast, or that they would give her a bottle of formula at the first opportunity if she wasn't feeding properly.

In fact, when Grace was finally born (in July 2006) after an exhausting twenty-four hours of labour, the midwife did push her face into me but I was too tired to be concerned. For the first two days, Grace seemed very reluctant to feed – I tried not to assume that she was now scared of my breast, as it was far more likely to be due to being drowsy from the drugs that I took during labour. I was really surprised that breastfeeding didn't seem to come naturally to either me or my baby. Holding her to my breast seemed awkward and uncomfortable, and Grace clearly hadn't studied the 'How to Breastfeed' photos of a baby opening its mouth wide to receive the nipple! She approached my breast more in the manner of someone about to suck a lemon. On the third day, the midwives started mentioning low glucose levels and, with the threat of the dreaded formula looming over us, I became even more determined to master breastfeeding and even stayed on an extra day in hospital to be sure I had the help I needed. I started asking for suggestions from every new midwife I saw in the ward, and became entirely unashamed about complete strangers grasping my nipple and shoving it towards Grace. My husband was as passionate as I was about breastfeeding, and it was wonderful to have his support at that moment when it seemed like it was never going to work. Finally I received two suggestions from a midwife which made all the difference. One was to imagine posting your nipple into a letterbox (squash it flat and push it in), and the other was to feed lying on my side. Grace fed for the first time once I tried these techniques in conjunction. I was jubilant about our first breastfeed, even if it was only for a few minutes, and finally felt ready to take our baby home.

My initial weeks at home with Grace were filled with manic charting of feeds and sleeps – how many minutes, which side, etc. I remember being quite hurt that the midwife laughed when I asked her how many minutes a baby should feed for in a day. I was just so concerned that Grace wasn't getting enough milk, as she would only feed for five minutes at a time before dozing off. Having read warnings about letting your child become a 'snacker', and that each breastfeed 'should' be at least twenty minutes to ensure the baby gets to the hindmilk,* I was desperate to get her to stay awake and have more. As such, I spent many a night taking all her clothes off and changing her nappy, holding her by open windows and so on, before finally being told by another health visitor that she might just be a very efficient sucker and that as long as she was putting on weight, I should stop worrying. That taught me to take all the advice in the books with a pinch of scepticism. A few other niggles arose over the following weeks, such as the fact that my back was hurting (a breastfeeding cushion sorted this out), that she wasn't latching on properly, and that as a consequence my nipples were very sore (lanolin cream provided blessed relief). But when Grace was around three months old, breastfeeding finally started to feel like second nature. I became incredibly glad that I had persevered – a feeling which lasts to this day – and was grateful that I didn't face any real difficulties. Quite apart from the well-known health advantages for both me and the baby, I've found breastfeeding to be convenient, comforting (to both Grace and me), and a great excuse to rest!

There's an unspoken rule amongst new mums that you don't comment on each others' parenting decisions, but that doesn't stop you making mental comparisons and knowing that others are doing the same. I remember, at an early reunion of our NCT class, that the one mum out of eight who wasn't breastfeeding made it clear that she thought we must think less of her because of it. It's hard to admit, but I was quite glad that the group who became my longer-term friends did all breastfeed their babies. Somehow, like my NCT classmate, I felt judged by all those who had taken a different route. I felt furtive when breastfeeding Grace in front of mums who bottle-fed, as though I was somehow showing off how virtuous a mother I was, or making a statement about what type of feeding I thought to be 'right'. I even resorted to saying self-deprecating things like "Oh, I'm just too lazy to bother with the fuss of bottles," as a form of apology for breastfeeding! It was therefore very reassuring to sit at friends' houses, all simultaneously breastfeeding without fuss or comment about it.

I did have a fairly obsessive attitude towards formula in the first six months, not wanting a drop of it to pass Grace's lips in case she decided that she preferred it. I was keen, however, to express milk so that my husband could have the experience of feeding Grace and so that I wasn't responsible for all of her feeds. She did take a bottle occasionally from about four weeks, but it was unfortunately short-lived. I found it very difficult to express unless my breasts were absolutely full, and I worried that I wouldn't have enough left if Grace wanted a feed. I was also frustrated that my electric breast pump made such a racket that it was difficult to do it when she was asleep. In the end, expressing became a chore which seemed unnecessary when I could breastfeed so easily. After a gap of a month or so between bottles, Grace decided that a bottle was something to be forcefully ejected from between the lips, and that was that.

The lack of bottle-feeding has been irritating to me at times – times when I would have loved my husband to take Grace with him for a few hours in the day (before she was weaned onto solids), or even now, to take a turn in the bedtime routine. On the other hand, I have been (still am!) fairly neurotic about leaving her with other people and I think I have unconsciously used the obligatory breastfeed as a form of control which has allowed me to stop enthusiastic grandparents from taking her away from me before I was ready.

I started to wean Grace on to solids at around five months, and dropped the mid-morning breastfeed altogether at around seven months. At nine months, I decided that I needed to move Grace onto milk from a cup during the day, in order to give myself more flexibility in leaving her with other people. Whilst I could have continued to mix breastfeeding and cup-feeding, I worried that this might confuse her so we switched to cup-feeding altogether for the afternoon feed. Just recently, around twelve months, I have started doing the same with her early morning feed. This was with some reluctance as I loved the half-hour that Grace, my husband and I spent in bed in the morning, but it was becoming incompatible with getting her to nursery two mornings a week. Grace has seemed entirely unconcerned at these changes, even though I have imagined her feeling as though I'm pushing her away from me. I find I often mix up my own feelings with those of my baby – she's a lot more independent than I give her credit for, I think. Luckily for me, Grace has recently started to give kisses and cuddles, so I get my emotional fix that way instead!

The only fly in the breastfeeding ointment has been some biting, which started as soon as she got her first teeth at six months. It was difficult not to shout in surprise, but this little display just delighted her and made her do it more often! I have since tried taking her off the breast when she does it and saying no firmly, and I think she does know that she's not supposed to do it now. But she still nips me occasionally and grins at my intake of breath, which makes her seem quite malicious! She's never bitten me so badly that I've been really hurt, although if she had I suppose it would have made me consider giving up breastfeeding.

However, after a year of breastfeeding, I can honestly say that it's been an overwhelmingly positive experience. It's made me feel deeply connected to my baby, and also to other mothers, it being such a worldwide, natural and ancient practice. I have, however, been quite surprised at the negative attitudes that I have encountered from family and friends who seem to see prolonged breastfeeding as slightly weird. Before the birth, my own Mum was quite vehement that I need not feel guilty if I couldn't breastfeed or if I wanted to give up early on (as she did with me). As I have continued to breastfeed Grace and clearly enjoyed it rather than finding it a chore, my Mum has continued to insist that I should "give myself a rest", telling me that I'll "have to give it up sometime", and gleefully pointing out that I'll have to do something about stopping now that I am pregnant for a second time. She may have felt that she's putting my welfare first and letting me know that it's OK to stop if I want to, but I've found this attitude a bit jarring as it's so at odds with my own. Other family members have made pointed comments about "Bitty" – a reference to a comedy sketch about a man who is still being breastfed in adulthood. Britain has one of the poorest breastfeeding rates in Europe, and I can't help but think that it is due to this pervasive attitude within our culture that breastfeeding is somehow a really taxing, and even distasteful, activity. Many mums seem desperate to get to the suggested six-month milestone so that they can stop feeding and get their body back to themselves, but I didn't feel that way. I hope that the new laws concerning breastfeeding in public and increased maternity leave will encourage and help more mums to start breastfeeding and continue for as long as they want.

So now, at thirteen months, we're just left with the bedtime feed. I am starting to regret that we've got into the habit of feeding to sleep, as it now seems an almost insurmountable obstacle to wean her off this feed. Whilst I would happily continue to breastfeed occasionally if that was feasible, I am at the point where I would like to share the bedtime routine with my husband and have the occasional night out. I therefore think it's best to wean Grace off the breast completely to keep consistency during the bedtime routine. At the time of writing, I am trying to get Grace to associate sleep with other things – lullabies, soft toys, stroking her hand. I'm putting off the first night when I don't actually feed her, and I know it's due to my own mixed emotions about giving up. I feel both privileged and proud to have breastfed Grace, and will now start to look forward to feeding my next baby – at least one of us will know what we're doing this time.

*****

Two years on and I'm happy to say that my second experience of breastfeeding was equally positive. I was a lot more relaxed about the process this time (as with most other aspects of parenting), listening mainly to my instincts rather than books or healthcare professionals. After a caesarean birth, it felt wonderful to revert to the natural practice of breastfeeding – to settle back into the familiar holds and latching technique.

When Laura was ten weeks old, however, I developed thrush. The shooting internal pains in my breasts made feeding excruciatingly painful, particularly at the point of latching on. One evening, when tired, stressed and extremely sore, I dug out the bottles and paraphernalia that I had kept from my failed attempts at expressing the first time around. Laura obstinately refused to take a bottle of formula – I'm sure she sensed my own reluctance. The ruling out of this alternative gave me the extra impetus I needed to grit my teeth and continue breastfeeding. I began to think that my familiarity with feeding had also led to me becoming lazy about ensuring a good latch, which was contributing to the pain. Once again I found myself looking for expert advice and found all sorts of tips and videos online. Focusing on improving my technique distracted me from the soreness, and within a week the worst of the symptoms had passed.

Laura and I then passed many months of contented feeding, and only when she was around fourteen months old did I start to think about giving up. I had learnt more about extended breastfeeding by this time, and was aware that it can continue without having to be part of a consistent routine. However, looking back at my diary, I think my desire to stop feeding Laura was tied up, subconsciously and rather irrationally, with wanting to spend more time with her older sister, Grace. In particular, I had missed reading her bedtime stories, having fallen into the routine of feeding Laura to sleep whilst my husband put Grace to bed.

I did worry about how both Laura and I would feel about finishing feeding (particularly in my case, because I was fairly sure that we wouldn't have another child). However, one evening my husband simply read some stories to Laura with a cup of milk, put her in her cot and, to our surprise, she went happily to sleep.

I felt (a little guiltily) that it was quite nice to be moving on from that generally exhausting first year. I breastfed Laura again one last time the following evening as a little farewell to that lovely phase of our lives, then simply stopped.

I continue to be a strong advocate of breastfeeding, and am so encouraged when I see Grace 'feeding' her baby doll under her jumper! I hope by the time my daughters are feeding their own babies that our culture will have changed to one where breast-feeding is accepted everywhere as a natural and healthy practice.

Alice's story

People asked me a lot when I was pregnant whether I planned to breastfeed. What I told them was that I planned to and hoped I would be successful. What I thought secretly to myself whilst giving this rehearsed answer was that there would be no way that I would fail at breastfeeding. It looked so easy after all. My Mum had breastfed me and my sister, all my friends with children were successful breastfeeders. I had dismissed the idea of bottle-feeding as inapplicable to me along with information about giving up smoking in pregnancy and domestic violence.

I planned to have my baby in a lovely midwife-run centre. I imagined myself sitting serenely in a birthing pool, listening to my birthing music CD. Unfortunately, the reality was somewhat different. I went into spontaneous labour when I was thirty-four weeks pregnant and my husband had to speed up the M62 to the nearest big city hospital. I found myself forced to lie on my back strapped to a foetal heart monitor as my son made his appearance into the world. He was handed to my husband for the briefest of moments before being whisked to intensive care to be helped to breathe. The midwife asked me if I had thought about how I wanted to feed my son and barely listened to my answer before announcing that he would probably have to be given formula until my milk came in.

I was taken down to the ward where I sat and waited for someone to come and see me. After five hours of waiting and being told that "someone would be coming shortly" about twenty times, someone appeared and told my husband that visiting times were over and he would have to leave. I panicked and said that if he was going then I was too. We signed the requisite forms and left the hospital.

I lay in bed that night reliving the day's events. I couldn't believe that my baby was here. Only hours before he had been inside me and now he was thirty miles away being cared for by a stranger. I didn't even know the way to the intensive care ward or who to ring to find out whether he was ok. I could almost believe that I had dreamt the whole thing.

The next morning we went to visit our son. Neonatal intensive care is a very bewildering environment, full of noisy machines, busy nursing staff and tiny, very sick-looking babies. Fortunately our son was doing well and giving the medical staff no real cause for concern. He was also not receiving any milk yet, but was on a drip instead. Whilst we were at the unit the midwife who had delivered our son appeared. She was horrified that I had discharged myself the previous night and had come to see if I was ok. She took me off into a side room and gave me an impromptu post-natal check. She also asked me if I had taken any action to get my milk going and gave me some advice about expressing some colostrum by hand. She found a member of staff and got her to show me where the hospital breast pumps were kept and how to connect them and express milk. The pumps were enormous contraptions on wheels which had the capacity to milk both breasts at once. Once you had finished expressing you took your little pot of milk and put it in a designated drawer in the room next door. I went to find my husband to help me with the process of extraction of the first few drops of my milk. I should add here that my husband is a vet and, I discovered, pretty knowledgeable about the process of milk production. He also has the ability to be totally unfazed by what some might consider embarrassing medical situations. I sat in an uncomfortable hospital chair while he rigged up the breast pump. I clamped funnels over both breasts and he switched the machine on. Nothing happened. Even the highest setting failed to produce any milk, so I set about attempting to express by hand, producing mere drops. Still, at least it was something. I trotted off to the freezer room only to meet another mother placing what seemed like litres in her drawer of the freezer. I resolved to ensure that my freezer drawer was full up as soon as my milk came in.

Armed with a breast pump I headed home and expressed every three hours around the clock. In the morning I would drive to the hospital with a cool bag full of little bottles of milk to be fed to my son through a naso-gastric tube. His requirements rocketed from 4ml every three hours to 30ml and I worried that I wouldn't be able to produce enough to keep up with him. One morning we went to the Special Care Baby Unit (he had been moved from intensive care by this point) to discover that he was being fed formula through his tube simply because the expressed breast milk in the freezer had run out and no-one had thought to phone me and ask me to bring in some more.

When my son had been in hospital for about two weeks we began to try breastfeeding. I found this very stressful. For a start he was not at all interested and just dozed away happily. I also had so much milk and got very uncomfortable after a couple of hours. I also had no idea about positioning and latching on. The ward was far from private and I sat behind a flimsy curtain with milk all over my clothes while nurses talked loudly about their weekend plans. Most of the other mothers whose babies were in special care weren't planning to breastfeed, although most of them had expressed milk for their babies at first.

After a few days of attempting to breastfeed my son during the day, I was asked by one of the nurses if I would like to come and stay in one of the rooms on the unit and try breastfeeding for forty-eight hours. If that was successful and my son was gaining weight, we would be allowed to go home. My husband unfortunately had to work for those two days so wasn't able to stay too. By this time I was finding feeding quite painful as my nipples were very sore. I soon started to dread my son waking up as I found the pain quite toe-curling. In hindsight I realise that I never really got my son properly latched on, but I lacked the confidence to say that something wasn't quite right. I asked the nurses for help and was told again and again that everything was fine. Eventually someone gave me some Lansinoh nipple cream, but even that didn't help.

At about 3am on the first night I was having terrible trouble getting my son to settle. I fed him and then lay him down in his cot, only for him to start screaming. Nothing seemed to settle him. I felt totally trapped in the room. I was desperate to take him back to the ward and leave him with the nurse and go home, but I knew that I had to prove that I could take care of him. I didn't feel like his mother at all; I felt totally unprepared to care for him. In desperation I walked down to the ward and asked one of the nurses for help settling him. The two nurses on duty that night were not particularly good English speakers and I had some trouble telling them what the problem was. They exchanged worried looks with each other and one of them said to me "You should go back to your room. If you ask for help then we will have to write on your son's medical notes that you are not coping". In tears, I walked back to my room and sat and cried, convinced that social services were going to be notified that I was failing to breastfeed. The nurse eventually came to my room and gave my son some of my expressed milk in a cup, which seemed to settle him. She told me that she was pregnant with her second child and was planning to bottle-feed.

In the morning I escaped from the ward and rang my husband

in desperation. He promised to come to the hospital as soon as he could. I went back and sat in my room with my son, who was now sleeping peacefully. After a few hours a nurse appeared at my door. She introduced herself as one of the community midwives and asked me how I was. I burst into tears and told her about the previous night. She was furious and said that if that happened again I should ask for the nurse in charge. She seemed very knowledgeable about breastfeeding and talked to me about it for a long while. I explained the problems I had been having the previous night with my son being very unsettled and she said she felt my son wasn't ready to try exclusive breastfeeding and should continue to be tube-fed for a few days. She then weighed him and her suspicion was confirmed as he had lost eighty grammes that day.

I went home to rest and woke up to discover that I had a blocked duct in my right breast, so increased my expressing and fortunately managed to clear it.

Several days later I went to stay at the hospital to try breast-feeding again and this time it was more successful. My son started to gain weight and seemed more settled. By this time my nipples were agonising, but I was determined to get us both out of there so I gritted my teeth. Finally, we were on our way home.

After a few days at home the pain in my nipples was so bad that I was crying throughout every feed. My husband trawled the internet for advice about latching on, but nothing we tried seemed to make any difference. I became so distressed that my husband made a decision to give our son some of my expressed milk (I had about six litres in the freezer) via a bottle. I decided that I would carry on with my expressing routine and bottle-feed for a few days to let myself heal. After doing this for a few days I realised that I had started to become dependent on knowing exactly how much my son was drinking each day and felt worried about going back to breastfeeding and the insecurity of not knowing whether he was crying from hunger or something else. So began my life of expressing and bottle-feeding. I continued to express every three hours around the clock.

Unfortunately I suffered repeated bouts of mastitis, which meant that my milk production dropped so much that I had to introduce one bottle of formula milk a day when my son was about two months old.

I continued this way for about four months until one day my son was screaming for his feed and his milk was still being defrosted. I was very engorged and needed to express and decided that, on a whim, I would try putting him to the breast. He latched on immediately and fed happily for some time. Feeding was a totally different experience this time round. There was no pain. I decided to try dropping the bottle-feeds one at a time and substituting breastfeeds and within two weeks we were back to exclusive breastfeeding. I did experience a little tenderness, but it only lasted a few days and was helped with Lansinoh and was totally different to the previous toe-curling pain.

When my son was about seven months old we went back to the hospital to a premature baby support group and saw the community midwife who had helped me. She had tears in her eyes when she saw that I had managed to breastfeed.

I stopped breastfeeding when my son was nearly eight months old. I had returned to work by this point and he refused to drink any expressed milk whatsoever, but would happily drink formula milk. I felt sad at the idea of giving up, but it wasn't possible for me to express at work and besides, I was totally sick of expressing at this point. Looking back, I am so pleased and proud that I managed to breastfeed in the end. It was the hardest thing I ever did, but also the best.

Di's story

Of course I'd never thought about breastfeeding before I was pregnant. Why would I? But once I knew I was expecting a baby, there was no question that it was the right thing to do. It's the most natural thing in the world and would give my baby the best start in life – I am fit and healthy and my baby would be too. The NCT class we attended was full of encouragement, which only confirmed that it is what I would do. I didn't buy bottles or a steriliser; there was no need as far as I was concerned.

The reality of trying to breastfeed when neither you nor the newborn know what you're doing is like sticking the tail on the donkey. The staff at the hospital where Molly was born were busy and unfortunately I felt a burden to keep asking whether we were doing it right. I remember the staff saying that I needed to make sure the whole nipple was in Molly's mouth otherwise I would be sore. I have to be honest and say that I'm not sure that they were that helpful.

We persevered though and when I got home my health visitor kept a check on us, offering tips and encouragement along the way. It was about a week after Molly had been born that I felt we had cracked it and we didn't have to think about it too much. Peter, my husband, made sure I ate properly as I had lost my appetite after the birth, which would not help with milk production.*

The intimacy that breastfeeding gave Molly and me is incredible – very special, private times, allowing our bond to develop into something that would last both of our lifetimes. This might seem over the top, but as I said it was incredible.

The staff at the hospital had been right, however, about Molly latching on properly. After about four weeks, I had a blister on my left nipple, which happened to be Molly's favourite breast. I had been confident that we were doing it properly because I could see her swallowing. She had been getting milk but still was not quite latched on with a good mouthful of nipple and areola. The blister caused me slight discomfort and more so when rubbing against my underwear. The health visitor soon realised what had happened and was able to correct our technique by watching us and giving us guidance. It didn't occur to me that I should stop breastfeeding, I just knew I needed to get the technique right. My first health visitor was incredibly enthusiastic and experienced and we all felt total reassurance from her visits.

I say first health visitor, as shortly after I had Molly, the allocation of health visitors across the region changed and I had a new one who was not quite as helpful. We then moved house and we were allocated a third health visitor!

It was hard for Peter as there was only so much he could do. I was feeding Molly on demand, which actually felt like all of the time. So we agreed that he would feed her in the evenings with milk that I had expressed earlier in the day. This would be one of my top tips, for two reasons. Firstly, it gave me a break and secondly Molly learnt to feed from a bottle – a different sucking motion and one that is forgotten if not kept up. This enabled us to have flexibility in who could feed Molly and ultimately allowed Peter and me to get out on our own.

When Peter and I decided to start a family we knew that we wanted two children, with a preference for them being close together in age if possible. Our understanding, from absolutely everyone, apart from one person, was that you need to continue to use contraception, whether breastfeeding or not. This we did in the first instance, as we wanted a small gap but needed to be sensible at the same time. After around four months, I went for a routine discussion with one of the GPs at my surgery. This was the one person who said to me "you won't get pregnant if you're breastfeeding". What a surprise (in that this contradicted what everyone else had said) and then what a dilemma. Should I stop breastfeeding Molly, potentially denying her of what I felt was the best thing for her, in order to conceive a brother or sister for her? We discussed it and decided on a compromise: carry on breastfeeding, but stop using contraception. We would take a chance on which advice was correct. I actually became pregnant two weeks after Molly's last feed, so you can make your own mind up![1]

I breastfed Molly until she was seven months old, which coincided with me going back to work. I had started to wean her by that point, and also introduced formula milk at around five months. I had been struggling to produce good quality breast milk and couldn't fill Molly up.* The first time I gave her formula milk I felt like I was giving her poison, but of course she was fine. She drank it and slept which meant I could sleep too and the quality of my milk returned.*

Weaning Molly meant she became less interested in my milk and we eventually got down to two feeds each day, morning and bedtime, until one morning I offered her a bottle instead and she took it without any fuss. We didn't breastfeed again after that, but I was positive Molly had had a fabulous start in life and she was ready for the next stage of mash, purée and plastic spoons.

I'm looking forward to breastfeeding my new baby when it arrives early in the new year. My thinking is that it is absolutely

---

1 Breastfeeding offers some contraceptive protection (and is used in some societies to naturally space pregnancies roughly three years apart, with important health benefits for both mothers and children – see Gabrielle Palmer's *The Politics of Breastfeeding* for more information on this). Dr Jack Newman describes the contraceptive effect of breastfeeding as being most reliable when the baby is under six months old, exclusively breastfeeding on demand (no bottles, even of expressed milk), and the mother's periods have not yet returned. Under these circumstances breastfeeding offers protection approximately equal to that of the use of condoms (around ninety-seven percent).

the right thing to do and is confirmed through a very positive experience. My sister's baby is due a couple of months after mine and I'm keen for her to try it too. I hope my determination to breastfeed and overcome any hiccups will rub off on her.

Louise's story

Of course I was going to breastfeed my baby. That's what all good mothers do isn't it!? There really was no question. Just like there was no question I would have a natural birth in a birthing pool with a natural expulsion of the placenta, gas and air for pain relief (epidural? no way!) and skin-to-skin contact immediately; just how my birth plan explained it.

So, my caesarean section was booked in for Monday morning… ok, so the birth hadn't gone to plan in any way (even doing hand-stands in the local swimming pool wouldn't turn my breech baby) but I was looking forward to breastfeeding. Maybe 'looking forward to' is the wrong expression – I'd had friends who had recently had children, one of whom just couldn't breastfeed despite all her efforts, and another who decided against it after six days of cracked and bleeding nipples. I wanted to breastfeed nonetheless, and was as prepared as I could be: I'd bought the nipple cream, knew of the cabbage leaf remedies should this not work, I'd read the instructions for both my breast pumps and had gone through the NHS leaflet on 'Feeding your New Baby' several times over.

Once my beautiful baby boy, Ashley, and I were wheeled into the recovery room, I asked the midwife if I could try to feed him. He seemed to be quite content lying there, but he didn't appear to be doing much, and it was difficult to get into a good position for feeding as I still couldn't feel anything from the chest down! So we decided to wait until I was in a position to feed him and he actually wanted to be fed.

The rest of the day was a blur of excitement with what seemed like everyone in our families cooing over the baby. Ashley started to get hungry, and our first night was an extremely long one... I can't remember how many times I tried to feed him that night but I was awake much longer than I was asleep! Each time I tried to feed him I pressed the 'alarm' button to request some help from a midwife – all of whom seemed to give me different advice on how to get Ashley to latch on and which positions to use. This was quite useful in some ways, as at least I was able to try a number of tactics. Sometimes I thought he was 'on' and feeding, and other times he obviously wasn't. I felt quite helpless after trying a number of times to get Ashley to feed, but the midwife reassured me that this was a skill that both myself and my baby would have to learn and it might take time and a lot of practice to get right. I was so relieved to see my husband the following morning. I couldn't believe how tired I was and it was only day one.

The next two days were tiring, with lots of attempts at breast-feeding, but Ashley didn't really seem to be satisfied for long. I didn't have any sensation of 'filling up' with milk, and even by day three, when most women's milk 'comes in', there was no noticeable difference. At this point, however, no one seemed particularly concerned that Ashley wasn't feeding properly; it was assumed he was getting enough. Later that day, Ashley was weighed and had lost fifteen percent of his birth weight – more than is normal (most babies lose up to ten percent of their birth weight then start to regain it again). At this point there was obvious concern that he wasn't feeding well. Various midwives monitored how Ashley was feeding, if I had him in the correct position and whether he was latching on properly. Although the actual breastfeeding felt painful to me at times, this didn't seem to be the issue according to the staff. A breastfeeding counsellor came to see me and asked me several questions, one of which was whether I had experienced any breast changes during pregnancy. The answer was no, I hadn't. This apparently can be one of the signs that breastfeeding may be problematic. I didn't know what to think – did this mean I wasn't going to be able to breastfeed? It was an upsetting thought as I hadn't even considered formula at this point. It was a lonely time as I didn't know what to do, was extremely tired, and Ashley was obviously very hungry! In the end the breastfeeding counsellor suggested a plan – we would cup-feed Ashley with 30ml of formula so many times a day, whilst I carried on trying to breastfeed as before (to encourage milk production), plus I was to use the hospital breast pump for a certain time after each attempted feed and if possible between 2am and 4am. Any milk that resulted from the pumping would be used as part of the 30ml feed, and this should increase day to day with the end result being no need for formula. This sounded exhausting, but encouraging, and I was willing to try anything! It was also a relief to be given 'permission' to feed my baby some formula, whilst I caught up with the breastfeeding.

The next few days were extremely difficult. The regime of feeding and pumping was exhausting. I seemed to spend every waking (and half-asleep!) hour either trying to feed Ashley or using the hospital's what seemed to be 'industrial strength' breast pump. (I soon switched to expressing by hand, as even though it was slow, it was much less painful). I really understood now what was meant by sleep deprivation. One night I remember being so tired after one of many middle-of-the night attempts at feeding, that I didn't have the strength to then use the breast pump. I picked Ashley up, walked to the midwife's desk and told them I couldn't do it any longer, that I was so tired I just couldn't face it. I burst out crying – it was all too much. There was so much pressure to keep up with the regime and my failure to do so was getting on top of me. My milk still hadn't 'come in' and I truly thought at this stage that it never would.

I had been filling in a feeding diary since it was recognised as a problem, and there would rarely be any longer than one and a half hours between my attempts to feed Ashley, especially at night, and feeds often lasted for an hour. Things gradually started to improve, however, and I got much better at hand expressing, to a point where I could actually gather enough milk for it to be worth trying to feed it to Ashley as part of his bigger formula feed. It was amazing seeing Ashley being cup-fed: he was lapping the milk up with his tongue like a puppy! It felt great to know that he was actually getting some of my milk now, and that soon I could hopefully feed him exclusively.

I left the hospital on day six, taking with me some cups for feeding and a couple of jars of formula. That evening we celebrated being home with a glass of champagne (whilst I was feeding Ashley – when was I ever not feeding Ashley?). I was happy to be home but nervous too, particularly about the feeding as there would be no midwife on hand for support or advice. That same evening a bizarre thing happened – my whole body began to shake. This lasted for about ten minutes and I had no idea what was happening. My husband was about to call the doctor when it stopped, and as I felt fine in myself we decided to put it down to exhaustion. The next morning, when the midwife visited to check all was well, she informed me that this is often a symptom of a woman's milk arriving. I can't explain how happy this made me feel – at last I was going to be able to breastfeed and might actually have enough milk to satisfy Ashley without having to formula feed him too!

The next few weeks weren't easy. Ashley still needed feeding a lot, noticeably (to me at least!) more than friends' babies born around the same time. I would dread night-times, going to bed as early as 8pm just to ensure I had some sleep before the seemingly endless night feeds began… it wasn't unusual for me to be sitting in the 'feeding chair' from around 11pm to 6am without actually going to bed. Ashley obviously wasn't feeding for all this time, but I would fall to sleep whilst he was feeding, then eventually, when I woke up and tried to put him in his cot to sleep, he would wake and be hungry again.

I remember one day when a health visitor came to see us, I'd had a particularly bad night with Ashley, was tired and (for the millionth time!) was considering whether it was worth carrying on breastfeeding. The health visitor said something that made me realise I would still be a good mum to Ashley if I decided to stop feeding him – as there was much more to being a good parent than simply breastfeeding your baby. Of course this was true; I just hadn't seen it like this before. Again, this was almost like someone's permission to stop breastfeeding, and I felt better to have this, even though I chose to carry on breastfeeding until Ashley was six months old.

I didn't feed exclusively for the six months. Apart from the formula supplements during the first couple of weeks, I breastfed exclusively until Ashley was two months old. I introduced a night-feed of formula at this point, as I felt (rightly or wrongly!) that I didn't have the amount of milk available that Ashley needed. Ashley would often be attached from early evening, around 5pm, to around 10pm, which signified to me that I wasn't producing enough milk for him.* Breastfeeding was constantly on my mind: why didn't I produce enough milk? Was the formula somehow damaging my baby? Why didn't I feel the 'let-down' reflex? Why did I seem to have so little milk compared to other mums? I decided to go to a breastfeeding support group, where I thought the other mums might reassure me that what I was doing was right. Instead, I was almost scared to mention the fact

I was supplementing Ashley's feeds with formula, and instead of supporting my decision, other members of the group just saw the formula as the problem and encouraged me to exclusively breastfeed. If I didn't already feel guilty about giving Ashley a nightly formula feed, I certainly did then (and, needless to say, didn't go to the group again!).

Health visitors would suggest Ashley was going through a 'growth spurt' and that by 'x' number of weeks things would improve and feeds would be quicker and more spaced apart. I carried on, believing that things must improve soon. They did, of course, but it took a while – at least a couple of months, and even then Ashley seemed to want feeding more than other babies his age. My weekly obsession with having him weighed proved that he was getting enough milk to stay on his line. I'm glad I stuck it out as I found breastfeeding to be the most convenient thing ever, and of course it's lovely to have that close time with just you and your baby. It was also nice to be able to relax for an hour whilst feeding in front of some mindless TV programme to try and recuperate from the previous night's missed sleep.

I learned some valuable lessons from my breastfeeding experience, and next time I will definitely want to breastfeed, but won't give myself a hard time if I find it too difficult to carry on (I can't imagine going through the same first few months I had with Ashley, with a toddler in tow!). My simple advice is just to enjoy your baby whether you carry on breastfeeding or not.

*****

My second baby was due on 14 October and my plan – as with my previous baby – was to breastfeed. Of course this time I'd have the benefit of experience; I knew how to breastfeed, but I also knew just how difficult I'd initially found it the first time. The health benefits and convenience of feeding made me just as determined to do it this second time round. Again, I'd had no noticeable breast changes during this pregnancy, so I was prepared for a re-run of what had happened with Ashley.

On 24 October I went into hospital to be induced – and to cut a long story short I actually achieved a normal(ish!) birth after two days of waiting and convincing hospital staff I didn't want another caesarean. My baby girl, Connie, was born on 26 October at 9.05pm. That first night in hospital with Connie was a bit of a blur, but I do remember trying to feed her without much success. Still, I'd been assured that this was fairly normal – lots of babies apparently need to rest, given the amount of energy used up during labour. The following day I fed Connie when she seemed to need feeding, although, as with Ashley, it didn't seem like she was really getting anything from me. But at least this time I knew how to latch her on.

After advice from midwives I began another regime of trying to feed Connie whenever she seemed like she needed it (a lot!) and expressing using the hospital breast pump in between feeds. It was exhausting but things did seem to be happening slightly quicker than they did with Ashley. I definitely wasn't as stressed out about it this time, as I knew that if I persevered then I could make it work. Still, being attached to a breast pump in the middle of the night whilst Connie was fast asleep, to achieve just a few millilitres of milk (if any!), was pretty disheartening. After a couple of days Connie was showing signs of dehydration and a paediatrician advised me (and the midwives!) that I'd need to 'top her up' with formula. Although I had wanted to avoid giving her formula, this was a relief (again!) to be given 'permission' to cup-feed Connie the extra milk she needed. I still carried on feeding her to the same extent as before (plus the expressing!), but she did seem to really need the formula top-ups. What I hadn't appreciated before was that if Connie was dehydrated she'd have less energy to feed from me, and as such she wouldn't stimulate the milk as much, so without giving her the extra energy she needed from the formula, she wouldn't have fed very well from me anyway. My plan, as before, was to reduce the formula cup-feeds over time to achieve her being fed exclusively by me.

The next two weeks were particularly tough, as every time we gave Connie a formula cup-feed I felt as if I wasn't doing what I was expected to do as her mother. I also felt bad for Connie as she was putting all this effort in to feed from me, but not getting what she needed in return – it hardly seemed fair. I often thought how much easier it would be to stop breastfeeding and put her on formula, but in my heart I knew what I had to do! We persevered and after just a couple of weeks I was feeding Connie exclusively.

During the following couple of months Connie woke at night every two to three hours for milk. I still didn't seem to be producing as much milk as I should, but she was putting on weight according to her 'line' on the weight chart. I again had a weekly obsession with weighing her at clinic, making sure she was getting what she needed from me. This was a good motivator for me, but friends with babies of a similar age just didn't seem to be breastfeeding quite as often as I was.

As the weeks and months went by things got much easier, with the gaps between feeds increasing all the time, except that Connie still seemed to need pretty much constant feeding between 5pm and 10pm for at least the first four months. At six months the time came to start weaning Connie – her first 'meal' was blended carrots mixed with baby rice (yuk!). As she was six months old I mixed the baby rice with full-fat cow's milk (I certainly didn't have the time to express for this purpose, and we had no formula in the house). I was surprised (to say the least) when within seconds of eating her first food, she came out in a red blotchy rash around her face and neck. Worried about the potential of an anaphylactic shock, crying, I rang the children's hospital to find out what I should do. They told me that if she hadn't had an anaphylactic shock by now then she wouldn't – it probably just meant that she was allergic to dairy. This was not great news. Obviously I wasn't to give her any more dairy products, and further tests revealed she was also allergic to egg.

What I hadn't realised at this point, was the effect this might have on my potentially stopping breastfeeding in the near future (I wasn't ready to stop just yet, but wasn't planning to breastfeed for too much longer). I didn't know that most formula is based on cow's milk and as such I wouldn't be able to switch her to formula. Apparently a couple of brands of formula are dairy-free, but they have an 'unusual' taste, or so our consultant told us. The consultant also mentioned that as Connie was breastfed, it was unlikely that she would accept the taste of such formula (breastmilk is very sweet-tasting). I was told, however, that from one year old (when it's possible to transfer a baby's main milk to cow's milk), she would be able to drink soya milk as a main drink. Apparently being intolerant to dairy is very common amongst babies, and given the chance to think it through this seemed quite logical: cow's milk (designed of course for calves) isn't necessarily going to suit a human being! This really brought it home to me how obvious it is that breast milk from a baby's mother contains exactly what that baby needs.

All this meant that I carried on feeding Connie myself, which I was quite happy to do. As she got older, feeds were quicker and further apart, and of course incredibly convenient (especially with a toddler in tow!). It got to the point where I was only feeding Connie in the morning, at midday (after her lunch) and in the evening, and eventually it was just morning and evening.

By the time she reached one year old I decided to carry on feeding her, even though at this point she could have soya milk instead – it was so easy and there was no washing of bottles or beakers involved.

At thirteen months Connie stopped breastfeeding on her own – for a few consecutive nights she'd been very fussy when trying to feed, and I'd noticed her nappies in the mornings were dry. From this point I started to give Connie soya milk in place of her breastfeeds – she accepted it straight away thankfully, and never even attempted to feed from me again. I didn't leak any milk at all, so Connie must have been reducing the amount of milk she'd taken from me for a while! Although it was sad to think I was no longer going to feed her, I was pleased she'd made the transition herself.

Rebecca's story

Before George, who is now nearly sixteen, was born, I hadn't given any thought to breastfeeding. At that time there wasn't as much emphasis on the benefits of breastfeeding and most of the information available related to formula feeding. I did look after a little boy who was breastfed when I was about fifteen, which was really the only image I had of breastfeeding. I was formula fed.

Luckily George was an absolutely brilliant feeder. He came out and fed straight away, latching on like a natural, even though I didn't even have a midwife to show me what to do. His was a difficult birth with forceps and ventouse and both he and I were quite battered and bruised. The feeding seemed to be the only thing that was going right.

George fed very efficiently – he would feed for ten minutes, sleep for two hours, then feed for ten minutes again. For the first six weeks he put on a pound a week in weight!

I had to have an operation under general anaesthetic when George was three months old. Up until that time he had been fully breastfed, but in those days they would not allow you to breastfeed if you were having a general anaesthetic and so he had to have some formula while I was operated on and in recovery.* After the operation I did continue breastfeeding but I was mix feeding with formula. He was fed half formula, half breastmilk until around six months when the formula took its toll on my supply and I stopped breastfeeding. My family had also been putting me under some pressure to bottle-feed.

I was sad to stop breastfeeding and I am a bit bitter with hindsight that the operation caused an early end to the feeding. If

I'd known then what I know now I wouldn't have allowed the operation to stop me fully breastfeeding.

Given how easy things were with feeding George, I was certain that I would breastfeed my second baby, Toby. But Toby was a completely different baby and an absolute nightmare to feed. He was relaxed and dozy at birth and never really took to feeding. He was born at 8lbs after a straightforward birth, dropped to 7lb 11oz and then didn't regain his birth weight for five weeks, a lot more slowly than the midwives and health visitors like to see. The health professionals were also concerned about Toby's health because he had only one artery and one vein in the umbilical cord.

To add to his slow weight gain, I was poorly after the birth. Some membranes that were left behind inside me caused an infection that meant I had to go back into hospital. Fighting off the infection and dealing with the hormonal changes going on in my body seemed to make it really difficult to concentrate on the breastfeeding and the chart in the 'red book' made worrying reading. It didn't help that the charts then were based on babies whose feeding was not differentiated – bottle-fed babies were included on the charts. I now know that Toby's growth would have looked different on the chart for breastfed babies.

My GP was suggesting formula, and my family were encouraging me to bottle-feed. My mother even sent me a newspaper cutting from America about a breastfed baby that had died, and encouraged one of her GP friends to tell me that my milk was 'weak'.

Toby obviously had other ideas, however, as he refused to take a bottle, and the single ounce of formula milk that we did manage to get down him was projectile-vomited straight back up. Fortunately I had a fantastic health visitor who came to see me every three days. If Toby had gained any weight at all in that time she would be happy and come back three days later. I also had a friend who was a breastfeeding counsellor who was very supportive and encouraged me to just keep feeding.

Fortunately, at around this time we took a week's holiday and my husband looked after George, which allowed me time to relax and just feed Toby. Things really started to improve at this point and in ten days he gained a miraculous 27oz!

If Toby had been my first baby, I'm sure I would have given up. But my experience with George meant that I knew how things could and should be, so I persevered through all the problems. Now Toby is much older I can see that his build is tall and slim, and he has a fast metabolic rate. He's very different to George, who is much stockier.

I fed Toby for sixteen months until he self-weaned. He dropped feeds until he was only feeding in the morning and at night, and the night feed, at about 11pm, was the last one to go. Once again I was sad to stop breastfeeding as it had been such a pleasure after the early difficulties. There's a real contrast here with parenting methods that encourage parents to drop night feeds as soon as possible – if I'd done that I'd have missed out on some really lovely time with Toby.

When Toby was eight months old I was contacted by the hospital, which was looking for mothers of eight-month-olds to volunteer to express milk for a baby who was ill in hospital and needed breastmilk to restore her gut flora. I and several other mothers provided expressed milk for several weeks until the baby was transferred to another hospital. It just goes to show how important breastmilk is for infant health.

By the time my third baby, Herbie, came along, I was confident and determined that nothing would get in the way of successful breastfeeding and I would not be derailed by health profession-als. Consequently whenever Herbie opened his mouth he got fed, and he never lost any weight. By twelve weeks he weighed 16lb 10oz! This time I took breastfeeding at my own pace and just enjoyed it – I never had any doubts or fears that things would go wrong. I would have argued the toss with any health professional who suggested I should stop or supplement.

Herbie, who's now four, can remember me breastfeeding him. Like Toby, he was around sixteen months when we stopped. He says that he can remember getting fed from my boobies and that he can remember the taste of the nice milk coming into his mouth. I'm fascinated to see what all three of my sons think about breastfeeding as they grow up and become adults and maybe fathers themselves. They've had so much exposure to breastfeeding that I hope they will all be thoroughly convinced of its benefits.

I co-slept with all three of my children and think that this really made night feeding easier and reduced our stress levels. I never had nights where I was walking the floor trying to settle them, and as the family grew it just seemed sensible that we all get as much sleep as possible. After all, I had to get up next day to look after the other children.

I'm saddened that women seem to have such a lack of confidence in their bodies – and their breasts – to do the job that they are designed for. It's also a pity that women who have themselves failed at or rejected breastfeeding feel the need to undermine women that are trying hard to make it work. I would say that breastfeeding can be hard but it is so rewarding that it is worth it. And the first six weeks are often the hardest. I wish women would allow themselves to just sit and feed in the early weeks – it's such a short time in the grand scheme of things.

Now that I'm a NCT teacher myself I've got a few pieces of advice that I would give to anyone: don't give up breastfeeding in the middle of the night – things can look quite different in the morning. If it's hurting, get some advice – it really shouldn't be painful. And don't be obsessed by the weight charts – all babies are different, and if you are getting plenty of wet and dirty nappies and your baby seems to be thriving, they probably are.

I loved breastfeeding my children and look back on it as a really pleasurable time.

I am beautiful as I am. I am the shape that was gifted. My breasts are no longer perky and upright like when I was a teenager. My hips are wider than that of a fashion model's. For this I am glad, for these are the signs of a life lived.

Cindy Olsen, co-owner of The Body Objective

I see my body as an instrument, rather than an ornament.

Alanis Morissette

Kirstie's story

Before the birth of my first baby, Ellie, I planned to try and breastfeed if I possibly could. Ellie was born in hospital in May 2005, after a very long and tiring labour. I was determined to try breastfeeding, but she wasn't so keen! On the postnatal ward I was told to wake her every six hours and try to feed. Ellie was more keen on sleeping and didn't seem that interested. I manually expressed precious drops of colostrum, which the midwives cup-fed Ellie for the first day. On the second day I decided I was just going to try myself, without help, and finally Ellie latched on. We didn't look back!

Ellie was a fairly contented baby, fed regularly and went for long periods through the night from an early age. I seemed to have an excess of milk, however, and wore breast pads throughout the whole feeding experience. The upside of this was that feeds were short and I could express a feed in five minutes flat. Ellie was quite happy to take an expressed feed and my husband enjoyed the experience of being involved in the feeding.

After weaning, Ellie carried on breastfeeding morning and night until she was a year old and then decided on her own that she wanted to stop. She has never drunk milk since, but gets her dairy intake with plenty of cheese and yoghurt.

Two years later when Edward was born peacefully at home, I didn't foresee any problems with breastfeeding. He breastfed straight away, but never stopped! His scream was high-pitched and made the glass in the house ring, and he fed so hungrily that I quickly developed very sore, painful nipples.

I was determined to carry on, and persevered through the pain. The feeds never seemed to satisfy Edward, and he would come off the breast red and screaming. He also refused to take an expressed feed, so I had no chance of a break. In desperation I tried dummies and formula – he refused both, and to stop the crying I put him back to the breast despite the pain.

Again, I seemed to have an excess of milk and so decided to express for the Milk Bank in Birmingham. This was extra work, but I was pleased to be able to make the contribution.

I looked forward to the milestones where I thought things might improve. Six weeks came and went and Edward was still unsettled. I decided it was colic and looked forward to the three-month milestone, but at four months he was still feeding at least every two hours during the night and, with a toddler to care for as well, I was exhausted. After consulting various breastfeeding books and websites, I cut the majority of dairy products from my diet, and at four and half months started weaning. Three

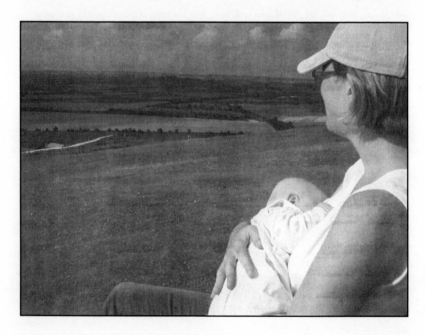

days later, Edward only woke once in the night for a feed and was smiling, laughing and like a different baby.

He is now almost five months old, and is much happier. I'm less tired, and breastfeeding is again a happy experience. I don't know what made the difference and whether it definitely was the exclusion of dairy from my diet, but for now I'm going to carry on with dairy-free breastfeeding.

I never expected breastfeeding to be so different between different babies. But just like their personalities, the feeding experiences are very individual.

A day came – of almost terrified delight and wonder – when the poor widowed girl pressed a child upon her breast... a little boy, as beautiful as a cherub. What a miracle it was to hear its first cry! How she laughed and wept over it – how love, and hope, and prayer woke again in her bosom as the baby nestled there... It was her life which the baby drank in from her bosom.

**William Makepeace Thackeray,
Vanity Fair, *Chapter XXXV***

The moment she had laid the child to the breast both became perfectly calm.

Isak Dinesen

Sophia's story

The year our baby girl was born via an emergency CS was a manic one. She was subsequently hospitalised at four weeks with blood in her poo. A few days after that, I sat and passed my medical exams. There was quite a lot going on so she was breast-fed and bottle-fed (formula or expressed milk).

She took to bottle-feeding quite well but, as the midwives told me, she was a 'lazy breastfeeder'.* I struggled to get her to latch on correctly. I used to refer back to the breastfeeding pamphlet we were given in hospital with the pictures of correct position-ing. My nipples were really sore. I used the yellow tube cream first of all but, I guess because it's a cream, it didn't work too well. I needed more of a Vaseline-type of cream. I switched to Lansinoh which really helped. I stopped using this at around eight weeks because one of my friends told me that thrush can thrive underneath the oily layer! I then used it every now and again, usually at night.

In the first instance, because I was revising quite hard, my husband took some time off and he always gave the middle of the night bottle. It was great to have that help as it gave me a straight five hours sleep (although I always woke up when she cried, at least I could go back to sleep). At six weeks my husband went back to work and my exams were over. We decided to exclusively breastfeed her, which in hindsight was the 'wrong' thing to do. We tried to reintroduce a bottle at eight weeks so that I could go off to have my hair cut, but she point-blank refused the bottle. I found that a similiar thing had happened with a couple of my friends when their babies were this age. At nearly five months old she started taking the bottle again – but only from me and only with those rubbery Nuk teats and warmed up.

I always said I'd give breastfeeding a go until six months and this is what happened – more or less. However, the road has been a rocky one. Apart from the pain that persisted up until she was around nine weeks old, which contributed to my lack of enjoyment of breastfeeding, she was also a very sicky baby. After every feed she would persistently bring up pools of clear fluid on our floors. However, she always put on weight. Looking back, I was feeding her every one and a half to three hours throughout the day and night – I guess to replace what she was losing. When she was about fourteen weeks old, I had a really bad night when she was so sick that I had to change my clothes three times and hers twice. I went to our postnatal group the next day and, looking around at the other babies, I realised that my girl was the only one with a bib on all the time, and when I burped her I had to be really gentle, whereas other babies were being quite vigorously burped – and without bibs! I went straight to the doctor's and she was diagnosed with reflux.

I kept a kind of breastfeeding diary:

Day one

First feed post-caesarean and I was really nervous. The midwife was fantastic, she just pulled out my boob and put my baby on. I needed her to do this as I couldn't move and was too worried that I wouldn't be able to bond with H because of the type of delivery.

Day two

Breastfeeding is really hard. I've had countless midwives helping me. Good job I get to stay in hospital for three days. Not sure how I'd ever tackle it otherwise, all the advice is invaluable. H is apparently a 'lazy feeder' although I have subsequently discovered that post-caesarean babies tend to be more sleepy.

Day three

Still haven't mastered 'latching on' and the actual feeding takes forever. Lying down is easiest.

Day eight

Breastfeeding in front of my friends as we revise together. In hindsight, this didn't help as I should have been paying more attention to the technique.

Day twelve

One feed can last up to fifty minutes. It's so tiring, but great for the weight loss!

Day eighteen

Had to feed her in the town centre on a bench today. No one seems to notice other than another mother who gives me a wry smile.

Day thirty

Met up with our antenatal group. It's interesting to see that most of the group are breastfeeding and on demand. No routines yet!

Day forty-nine (seven weeks)

It's still painful and I keep checking my technique. Just want to get to eight weeks and then I might switch to the bottle. I really don't like breastfeeding much but I know it's good for her.

Day fifty-six (eight weeks)

I think H and I are just starting to get in tune with each other. It's starting to hurt less and I'm using less cream. Tried the bottle again just so I can go out for a few hours, but she's not having any of it.

Nine weeks

It hurts just for a bit every time I start feeding her, but with the correct positioning, tummy to tummy, that seems to have done the trick. Feel the milk coming out of the breast, like a tickle.

Twelve weeks

Nightmare time with feeding her. She's feeding on demand every one and a half hours at night, but every three hours in the day. She's so sick as well. Having to use the cream a bit again as my nipples are so sore.

Fourteen weeks

Reflux diagnosed and Carobel started.

Seventeen weeks

She's finally slept right through one night, yippee.

Eighteen weeks

She's jumped up a centile in weight now she's holding down her food and I'm now in a routine with her, as on-demand feeding doesn't work when Carobel has to be given before every feed. I'm slightly envious of the other girls who can feed on demand, it's so much more in tune with the baby's needs. However, now her reflux is better, I can deal with routine!

Twenty-one weeks

Started weaning her onto the bottle. Starting with the bottle and finishing with the breast in order to reduce my milk supply. Going really well since someone told me that breastfed babies like their formula milk warmed up. Decided not to express as it increases milk production and I won't be expressing when I return to work. I'm finding it really hard emotionally to swap her onto the bottle. I've had a good cry and really surprised myself. I always thought it would be easy to stop breastfeeding but I feel like every time I give her a bottle it means she doesn't need me any more. Crazy considering the number of times I wanted to give up!

Twenty-one weeks and three days

Unfortunately, her sickness is coming back and she's very windy. This evening she was in real pain as it kept coming back up whilst she tried to go to sleep. I'm going to have to change my game plan. Back to breastfeeding and weaning onto solids instead then onto the bottle or even a sippy cup in a month's time. Tomorrow is going to be hard work as my milk production will have decreased.

So there we are. My breastfeeding story. Having been so adamant that I would never breastfeed beyond six months, I suspect that if it wasn't for my imminent return to work at seven months, then I might just carry on until she weans herself. I hated breastfeeding initially, found it painful for weeks but once I'd cracked it (probably a lot to do with position as well as her reflux issues) then I've grown to really enjoy it. It's a lovely feeling to see her staring up at me and chatting once she's finished. She also pats my breast and strokes my skin which is adorable.

When she first felt her son's groping mouth attach itself to her breast, a wave of sweet vibration thrilled deep inside and radiated to all parts of her body; it was similar to love, but it went beyond a lover's caress, it brought a great calm happiness, a great happy calm.

Milan Kundera

Ah, the joy of suckling! She lovingly watched the fishlike motions of the toothless mouth and she imagined that with her milk there flowed into her little son her deepest thoughts, concepts, and dreams.

Milan Kundera

Sarah's story

My daughter Harriet was born after an easy, positive labour and birth. She latched on soon afterwards which was wonderful and seemed to be just the right thing. For the next two months she fed well and I quite enjoyed the experience. She was an extremely sicky baby and I felt as though I was always covered in milk and vomit and never left home without a stash of muslins! Between her second and fourth months she slept fairly well at night, but during the day she fed every hour. I could not do a shopping trip without having to feed her in the checkout queue! I am sure that she was vomiting half of most of her feeds which didn't help. So at four months I took her to the doctor who prescribed Gaviscon to help with the sickness. Although this did help it was quite difficult to use as it involved expressing milk to mix it with and spoon-feeding her with it as she would not take a bottle. I only used it for the first feed of the day but found that things were better for the next two or three feeds. At this stage I also started weaning. She became a much happier and more contented baby overnight. I felt as though I had been starving her for the previous eight weeks. After perseverance she started to take a bottle so at four and a half months I introduced a bottle of formula once a day which she took well. A month later I introduced the second bottle at which point she decided that she would rather bottle-feed than breastfeed.* Although I felt guilty about it as I had been planning to breastfeed for one year, my predominant feeling was relief as it had been a stressful, over-whelming experience. I was very lucky to have been very well supported to breastfeed. My mother, mother-in-law, sister and husband are all very pro-breastfeeding, which did help. I also have many friends who breastfeed their babies, and I think there is a lot to be said for going to a breastfeeding support group.

Lots of people told me that having a second baby would be easier. "How is that possible?" I thought, "When I will have a toddler to look after as well?" I anticipated another stressful first few months, but never considered doing anything other than breastfeeding as I still strongly believed in the health benefits for myself and the baby. I planned to get to six months when I felt it would be acceptable to stop. Again I was lucky enough to have another very good birth experience, this time at home. Eddie fed within an hour of birth and latched on very well. He seemed to have a much stronger suck than I remembered Harriet ever having. He was a little bit sick every now and then, but nothing like as much as Harriet had been. He fed fairly frequently and for the first ten weeks he had a three-hour sleep every lunchtime which really took the pressure off me. I was also pleased to have

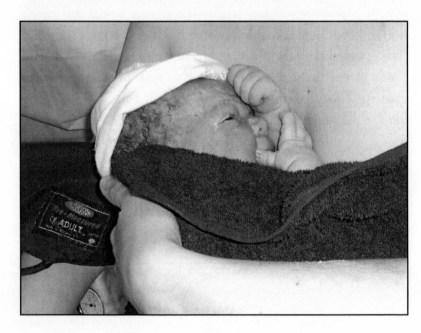

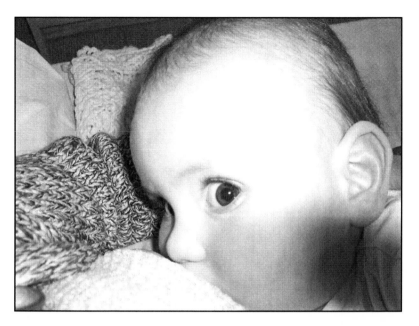

a bit of a routine, as this had not happened with Harriet until after I had stopped breastfeeding. He was a very happy contented baby in a way that Harriet had not been until she was much older. At fifteen weeks he suddenly stopped sleeping well at night, started to feed constantly and was miserable most of the time. I had hoped to make it further than four months before starting to wean him, but it was not to be.* Things improved very quickly and we had our smiley happy boy back. However it went from one extreme to the other as he started to have very short, infrequent feeds. I worried about this quite a bit and found the staff at the local breastfeeding group and several friends very encouraging. A good friend said that the same had happened to her and that he had probably just become a super-efficient feeder.

He has just reached six months now and in the past two to three weeks we have managed to have a regular breastfeeding routine. Four feeds during the day and one at night. He sometimes sleeps through and I'm sure that if I tried to comfort him instead of feeding him he would probably give up the night feed, but strangely I don't want to. I am enjoying breastfeeding so much this time that I would like to do it for a year or longer. I have a feeling though that Eddie might have other plans!

Anna's story

Before I gave birth I knew that I wanted to breastfeed. I'd already looked around town at places I knew were breastfeeding-friendly for feeding in public, and friends had given me advice about feeding discreetly with a muslin over one shoulder.

When Jake was born it took some effort to get breastfeeding established. I didn't get chance to feed Jake within the first hour of his birth because I was transferred from the midwife-led birth centre where he was born to hospital in an ambulance because of a retained placenta. Jake didn't really latch on at all for 36-48 hours after birth, although I tried a lot of different positions. He was quite sleepy and not very interested at first.

I transferred back to the midwife-led centre for post-natal care and was there for three days. I was determined not to leave before breastfeeding was properly established. I had advice from a variety of different midwives, who each had their own approach: more mature midwives seemed more keen to grab hold of my boob and try to latch Jake on, while the younger ones were keen to get me to try to latch him on and made suggestions including expressing a little milk first to soften the breast. Perseverance and trying different things eventually worked and we went home.

Once home and having visits from the midwives I got better advice, including using hot flannels to help with engorgement and recommendations to empty one breast fully before switching to the other. Jake took a long time to feed and the midwives said this didn't matter – you have to go with the speed of the milk flow and the demands of the baby in the early stages to get feeding established.

After the first week or so I would get a kind of toe-curling pain just when Jake latched on – for about ten seconds or so. I met a school friend in Asda who'd had the same thing and reassured me that it was like breaking in a new pair of shoes! She was right and soon this pain disappeared.

I fed on demand the whole time and in the beginning this meant very long feeds indeed and I had to organise my life around feeding and just go with what Jake needed. Sometimes I did need to interrupt his feeds and I found this quite upsetting.

At four months Jake was noticeably taking more milk and I was feeling tired. At about five and a half months I started weaning and, as his intake of solids increased, he soon got into a routine of four feeds a day. At six months we introduced one bottle of formula at night. He'd had expressed milk in a bottle prior to this, but only intermittently. This was partly in preparation for me going back to work when Jake was six and a half months old.

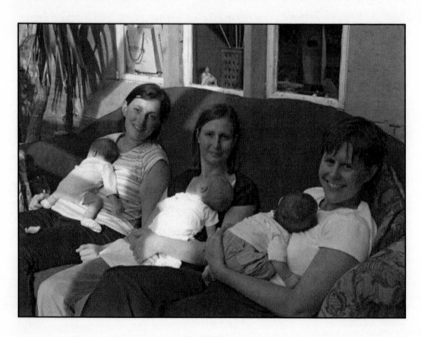

When Jake was at nursery I breastfed him in the morning, when I picked him up from nursery in the early evening and at night. At the very beginning I expressed milk for him to have in a bottle while at nursery, but it was difficult to find the space and time at work to do this and he soon went on to having formula milk at nursery and me the rest of the time. I continued to feed him more at the weekends and when I wasn't at work.

When Jake was nearly a year old I was away from home for three nights. He had bottles of formula while I was away but I expressed milk to keep my supply up and just went back to feeding Jake as normal when I got home.

While teething Jake did pull off and cause me real pain a few times, but he learnt to hold the nipple differently once he had teeth and it did improve. For a few weeks he also used to get very distracted while feeding, which sometimes led to him pulling off, and I fed him in a quiet room for a while until the phase passed.

By the time Jake was a year old I was still breastfeeding and not feeling at all like stopping. At around this time I did begin to feel a bit of pressure to stop and it seemed as if even those people who were being supportive were now doing so by saying "it's alright to stop". My mum said "you have been doing it a long time". We were going away on a holiday and I had always thought it would be easier to be breastfeeding for that trip. I fed Jake even more than usual while we were away and I did notice the difference that made to me physically – I was certainly more tired.

I kept expecting my milk to dry up naturally and the fact that it didn't made me feel like my body was designed to carry on breastfeeding.

When Jake was fourteen months I gave up the morning breastfeed and Graham, my husband, gave Jake some milk in a cup instead. To start with this was very difficult as Jake would be angry and I would lie in bed listening to him cry and getting very upset myself. We kept going with the night feed for another month and this proved much easier to drop. Until then I had been feeding Jake to sleep and I was worried about how he would settle without it, but he was fine. By this point it seemed as if giving up breastfeeding was a bigger thing for me than it was for Jake!

Overall I would say that breastfeeding Jake has been a wholly positive experience and I'm proud to have done it for so long. Since stopping I've found that some of the joint pain and achiness I'd been having while breastfeeding has improved. I also used to find that the long night feed, although a lovely time for Jake and me, was a real responsibility and I can now share that with Graham, which gives me a new freedom. I'd say to any new mum that the easiest way to breastfeed successfully and keep going is to be as relaxed as possible and just go with the flow – the more you try to control things, the harder it gets. Supportive friends are really helpful and can give you the confidence you need in the early weeks: we went to see friends in Kent when Jake was very small and Chris, a male friend, helped me latch Jake on in a restaurant in front of the other diners and his relaxed attitude really put me at ease.

Helen's story

When I learned that I was expecting twins, I immediately knew that I would feed them myself. I'd breastfed my first son until he was fifteen months old and felt that I knew what I was doing. I expected to face some challenges with feeding twins: the usual struggles with latching on in the early days, and wondering about the best holds – but the reality turned out to be very different.

I had an elective caesarean section because 'twin one' was breech. My son had been a 9lb baby, and when the twins were delivered at thirty-four weeks they were already around 6lbs each. They were both in good shape at birth and didn't need any help with breathing or other special care. Fortunately they both had a sucking reflex and were able to latch on. In retrospect I was shocked to think that when we were discussing when the twins should be delivered, no one mentioned to me that they could have lacked the sucking reflex at thirty-four weeks gestation. If I had known that this was possible I might have been keener to wait a little longer before having the section, as I would not have wanted to jeopardise my chances of feeding them successfully myself.

I remember being asked, as I was given the epidural in theatre before the babies were born, how I intended to feed the twins and replying that I definitely intended to breastfeed them.

In the early days my baby girl, Nova, was very sleepy and reluctant to feed. She was weighed by a midwife a couple of days after we'd gone home and she had lost around ten per cent of her birthweight. We were not concerned about her, but the midwife 'gave' us a couple of days to 'sort it out', threatening us with readmission to hospital if her weight gain didn't improve.

I had some advice from a lactation consultant on an internet forum that I use regularly, Mumsnet. She had breastfed twins herself and I found her advice very helpful. She suggested that I should tell the midwife that I had spoken to a lactation consultant and that I should then ask the midwife about her own experience in supporting breastfeeding, if I felt that the midwife was being too over-zealous about Nova's weight.

In the course of my research I learned about the technique of breast compression, which can help sleepy or slow feeders to take more milk at each feed and improve slow weight gain, among other benefits. I used it with Nova to great effect.

Next time the midwife came to weigh Nova, she was still concerned about her weight. She was even talking about calling a paediatrician and readmitting her to hospital, which we felt was unnecessary. In the end she agreed that I could feed Nova and that then we would weigh her again, which I agreed to even though I knew that this is a poor way of measuring weight gain and was thus a pretty pointless exercise. So I fed Nova, using the breast compression technique, and the midwife was astonished at the results. Nova immediately weighed considerably more, at which point the midwife exclaimed that if I had only fed her before she arrived, she would never have had cause for concern.

From the start I fed the twins individually, rather than at the same time (tandem feeding). I never really had a problem with them both screaming to be fed at the same moment – I was demand feeding and would start to feed as soon as I picked up on the cues from one twin. The other would usually be happy to wait since they were some way off screaming to be fed. Occasionally they would coincide and at those times I did tandem feed them. I felt that feeding them individually helped with the bonding process and enabled me to establish individual relationships with them.

When tandem feeding my baby boy, Dante, would put Nova off feeding as he was fussy and difficult. He was very unsettled and wanted to feed constantly. Nova was always the better sleeper, and she still is now.

Dante's problems with feeding meant that, when he was three or four weeks of age, I found myself searching 'vomiting through nose' on the internet. He would suddenly go bright red and scream, would vomit a lot and would cry inconsolably with gastric pain. I took him to the doctors and we were immediately diagnosed with reflux problems and put on infant Gaviscon, which was a pain to administer to a breastfed baby, and Ranitidine. Unfortunately the medication made no difference to his symptoms, and it was only after I came across the possibility that dairy products in my own diet were the cause (thank you Mumsnet) that I was able to try an exclusion diet. Within three days of cutting dairy out of my diet, Dante's symptoms vanished. He began to pile on weight and was much more contented.

At about this time I started to find blood and mucus in my daughter's nappy. She became more unsettled and was having eight or nine dirty nappies a day, which my instincts told me wasn't right for her. I took her to the doctor's several times but they weren't really interested. They sent off a stool sample which didn't show anything, and offered hydrocortisone cream at the third visit. I even got that old chestnut 'Is this your first baby?' However, my experience with Dante encouraged me to do my own research into 'food-induced proctocolitis', and in the next few weeks and months I found, by elimination, that Nova was allergic to fish, soya, gluten, dairy, pork and eggs. My own diet had to change considerably. I eat a lot of potatoes, rice, chicken, pulses and fruit and vegetables – treats include chips and plain, dark chocolate. IBS symptoms that I had experienced myself cleared up.

Because I knew about the twins' allergies, I was able to wean them onto foods I knew that they could tolerate. When, at nine months, I offered them a sip of goats milk that led to inconsolable screaming and a rash, the doctor finally referred us to a specialist for a full range of allergy testing for the twins, and advice from a dietitian for me.

The twins are still breastfed and have no other liquids. I am expressing milk for them on the days that I work. Under the supervision of the specialist we are going to trial them on hypoallergenic formula to see if they can tolerate it – although it is based on cows' milk it is extensively hydrolyzed and may not cause symptoms, although it does taste vile and is expensive.

I intend to feed the twins until they wean themselves and it has never occurred to me to give up – the alternatives have never seemed to offer any benefits, to either the twins or me. I've found breastfeeding them, and getting to the bottom of their allergy problems through my own research and testing, to be a tremendously positive and empowering experience. I've trained to be a peer supporter of breastfeeding and think that through this, and website communities such as Mumsnet, women can really help each other by sharing their knowledge. I feel a responsibility to help correct the duff advice that so many people are given about breastfeeding, from their friends and family as well as health professionals. So many breastfeeding relationships could be saved by better knowledge and advice, less intervention and more peer support. When my first son was born I went to a drop-in breastfeeding clinic where every week a new mum would turn up and need support from those of us who'd been there longer. I went for six or seven months and loved the way women were helping each other out just by getting together.

In all the time I've been breastfeeding the twins, the attitudes of other people towards me have been the same: everyone is amazed that I have done it and kept going so long. One health visitor told me that in eight years of practice she had never met a mum who had successfully fed twins. A GP asked me if I had enough milk, and a midwife in hospital seemed almost put out when I refused to take advice about cup and syringe feeding and expressing milk, preferring to get straight on with getting the twins breastfeeding normally. The consultant who delivered the twins told me "you have to impose your will on twins, you know" – which I also ignored, feeding them on demand right from the start. A colleague at work is quite opposed to breast-feeding and has asked me why I don't just pack it in, which I find baffling as I can't see why I would want to!

My family have been very supportive – my own mother breastfed three children and has a real 'can do' attitude, and my partner has been really, really supportive and is a total advocate of breastfeeding. His family had little experience of breastfeeding but have also been supportive.

No one could give her such soothing and sensible consolation as this little three-month-old creature when he lay at her breast and she felt the movement of his lips and the snuffling of his tiny nose.

Leo Tolstoy

[How long did you breastfeed Jaden?] *A good 18 months. That baby never even saw a bottle. He went everywhere with me — premieres, award shows. I would just find a back room and hook him up.*

Jada Pinkett Smith

Jen's story

NB: *Jen is in the US*

Breastfeeding has always made perfect sense to me, so when I found out that I was expecting Eamon, I knew for certain that I would breastfeed him; it was a given.

I feel that my upbringing had a great deal to do with shaping my feelings about breastfeeding: I am seven years older than my brother and have only much younger cousins. As a young girl, I witnessed my mother and my aunts breastfeeding their babies. I can honestly say I have no memory of any woman in my family ever using a bottle.

Once I realized I was having a baby I went out and bought every book on the shelves regarding pregnancy, birth and the first year. My reading confirmed what I already knew: that breast-feeding was the best start for the baby. The choice to breastfeed also seemed natural to me given my lifestyle – I practiced yoga including prenatal, tried to exercise daily and had basically a vegetarian diet. I was planning on having a 'natural' labour and delivery, that is to say no drugs, and thought that I would breast-feed exclusively from the start.

Well… my best-laid plans quickly went out the window during my labour… it was long and agonizing and I desperately accepted any sort of medical intervention that would save me from the horrific contractions. After thirty-six hours of labour I had no dilation to speak of, the baby had passed meconium and his heart rate dropped hazardously low on two occasions. The doctor said it was time for a C-section. Although I was eager for the baby to be born, I felt, even at that moment, like a huge failure since I was not able to have a vaginal birth.

Soon after Eamon was delivered, examined and washed up, they placed him between my legs and wheeled us up to our room. He was a healthy, big baby who didn't appear to suffer too much given the stress he went through and subsequent C-section birth. I, on the other hand, was a mess given the lack of sleep, interventions, and operation. Still, I was determined to breast-feed. With the help of my nurse, I held him to my breasts, and he began to feed vigorously. But subsequent feedings proved more difficult. I was feeling so nauseous from the post-op meds that I would have to quickly stop feeding him in order to vomit. My nurse made the extremely inappropriate comment, "Maybe something Freudian is going on". Clearly this was not the beginning to breastfeeding that I had imagined.

My three-night stay in the hospital proved equally trying. The night nurse came in around midnight to take Eamon for his nightly check-up. When she brought him back to me she demanded, "What are you doing with this baby, he's lost a lot of weight!". I started to cry. Soon after, two other nurses came in and strongly 'suggested' that I introduce formula since, in their opinion, he was clearly not thriving with breast milk alone. Again, feeling like a failure, I gave in to this request, thinking that they knew best. I remember them offering Eamon formula in a little tiny cup and him lapping it up like a kitten. I felt extremely uncomfortable with this but again reasoned that the nurses knew best. Well, no sooner did they leave the room than Eamon started vomiting up the formula. From that moment on I swore that I would not use formula again and first thing in the morning I was going to request a lactation consultant.

In retrospect, asking for a visit from the lactation consultant was one of the first steps I took in taking control as a mother. This woman was fantastic. She explained how normal it is for babies to lose weight during the first few days and that introducing formula was not necessary. She marched over to my bed, lifted up my pajama top and, not at all gingerly, placed Eamon up to my breast. He started to feed like a pro and she declared, "there's nothing at all wrong with you or the baby; continue breastfeeding!"

This was extremely encouraging and was the first boost of confidence I received from anyone in the hospital.

In the weeks that followed, I struggled with negative feelings of being a "failure" with the birth. The one thing that kept my spirits up, however, was the success we were experiencing with the breastfeeding. It became more natural with each passing day and I was so proud to learn of Eamon's weight gain at his first week doctor's visit.

I continued to breastfeed Eamon, on demand, until he was about twenty-two months and I was in my second trimester with my second child. At that point, breastfeeding was becoming painful and I felt that I wanted a bit of a break between my first and second babies! Although I was keen to wean Eamon, he was not so keen and I turned to a breastfeeding support center for help. The woman offered me the advice, "don't offer but don't refuse". I adopted her advice and this got us down to one feeding at night before bedtime. The last feeding occurred transatlantic as we were flying back from London to New York. As I was breastfeeding Eamon (while squished in a plane seat) it became so painful that I actually saw stars! I turned to my husband and proclaimed, "This is it: I'm done with breastfeeding!". Luckily enough, Eamon didn't seem to mind. The next couple of nights, he made a couple of half-hearted attempts at bedtime. However, when I didn't readily cooperate, he quickly gave up and forgot about it.

I had about a five-month break from breastfeeding Eamon before I gave birth to my second child, William. Although I wound up having him via C-section as well (despite my best efforts to give birth 'naturally' it wasn't meant to be), I had much more confidence with his arrival and did not hesitate to begin and continue breastfeeding. At thirteen months William is still successfully breastfeeding and I have no plans to wean him until we are both mutually ready.

Zoe's story

We gave birth to our son in December 2005. Throughout the pregnancy and our preparation breastfeeding the baby was something that we wanted to be able to do. We had a number of positive messages around us that helped with this. Both of our mothers had breastfed their children (we are each one of three) and were quite happy to talk about their experiences, positive and negative, and they were also supportive of us breastfeeding if we could but also didn't put pressure on us. One of my sisters is a nurse and had recently undertaken the national Baby Friendly breastfeeding course, my other sister was pregnant and was wanting to breastfeed, and we also undertook the NCT classes in the last few weeks of pregnancy.

As often happens, Daniel's birth didn't quite go to plan. We had wanted a hospital-based water birth with low/no pain relief, but he was overdue so we had to be induced and I ended up having all the pain relief available and just achieving a natural delivery. He came out a large 9lb baby – who actually looked more like he was three months old! We tried to initiate feeding in those first few hours, but he wasn't interested and just wanted to sleep. He was born in the early hours of New Year's Eve, so the fireworks about eighteen hours later for the start of 2006 woke him up and it was at that time we had our first feed. Latching on didn't seem very straightforward – but as the ward was quiet I had one of the midwives sitting with me for well over an hour and eventually we achieved it. However, reality really kicked in about thirty-six hours later when my milk properly came in. I had already discharged us home by this point. I woke up from a sleep feeling like I had two watermelons strapped to my chest. I am big-breasted anyway (34FF) and I couldn't believe how much bigger I had got, I actually needed help sitting up! The community midwife did her first home visit that day and tried to encourage me to feed Dan in the rugby ball hold position. It just didn't work, we were both far too big and I couldn't hold Dan for the length of time needed without feeling strained and uncomfortable. So we reverted to the normal hold.

Feeding started to settle in. Dan would feed for quite long periods of time (thirty to fifty minutes) but once satiated we were soon going four hours between feeds, which helped us all from a sleep point of view. We had also decided that we would take the opportunity to introduce the bottle into feeding so that David could have a more active role with Dan – particularly at bedtime (I still took the night-time feeds). Whilst Dan wasn't too sure what to do with the teat at first – he kept rolling it around with his tongue – he soon grasped it and David loved being able to feed him.

This helped with the 'big decision'! My youngest sister was due to get married in South Africa at the beginning of April when Dan would be about twelve weeks old. Neither me nor my sisters could imagine me not being there for the wedding, but neither could I imagine the new family making the journey. After much soul-searching we decided that I would go to the wedding – for the shortest time period physically possible – and David would stay at home with Daniel with the support of his parents. The planning began! I was to fly out on the Friday morning, arrive in South Africa early that evening, attend the wedding on the Saturday and fly home Sunday afternoon, physically getting home on Monday at lunchtime.

We wanted to continue Daniel on breast milk as much as possible. The time away translated into feeds required a freezer stock of 125 fl oz of breast milk. We put a plan together which meant 5 fl oz being expressed on a daily basis. It was frozen in a mix of sizes (1-5 fl oz) so that any size of feed could be made up, and we stored it in two or three different freezers in case of mechanical failure. I must admit there were some days when I felt more like a cow with my automated breast pump – but it was one of my ways of reconciling with myself that I was going away. We also started giving Dan the very occasional feed of formula so that we knew whether he would take it and that we had a further back-up plan if needed. We also increased the number of feeds he had from the bottle and included David's parents in giving him his feeds.

I also sought out one of the breastfeeding advisers in the city so that I could talk it through with her – one particular area of concern was whether having a particularly prolonged period of bottle-feeding would interfere with being able to go back on the breast. The adviser was incredibly supportive and very pragmatic. She didn't think there would be a problem, but said that we might have to do a little relearning, and offered her support and direct contact number if I needed increased input on my return.

The wedding weekend came and David's parents moved in. Leaving the house with David's dad for the airport was just awful but it still felt the right thing to do.

The reception in South Africa from my sisters and mum when I got there proved that and the wedding was beautiful. I kept up with expressing milk throughout the weekend, finding that I wasn't producing as much as I thought I would, and struggling with the concept of tipping it down the sink – but I really enjoyed myself.

I got back to David and Daniel. Everything at home had gone completely to plan. Dan and I quickly settled back into breastfeeding and our routine continued.

One particular feature of Daniel throughout his breastfeeding time was his irregular poo cycles! We did find it rather concerning and it was one area we sought advice over. Early on he stopped pooing on a daily basis and moved to going anywhere between two and five days. It just didn't feel right. However, what we got back was consistent advice from our health visitor, the breast-feeding adviser and agreement from our GP, which was this: sometimes breastfed babies are so efficient in their use of the breast milk that they produce very little solid waste. Everything else with Dan was fine – he was gaining weight, he was produc-ing wet nappies, he was still going four hours between feeds and sometimes longer, including up to nine hours during the night. Nonetheless, it was still something we struggled to reconcile and also, when he did go, it tended to be quite a volume and rarely stayed in the nappy (thank you to anyone who either witnessed it or helped on one of the clean-ups!). Daniel was not at all distressed during this period – he had no signs of tummy ache, he tended to be calm when he was going – but it did mean that the more days 'without' meant me going everywhere with at least one towel, extra clothes, wipes and so on, and Grandpa being ready with the jet wash if he supervised Dan whilst I popped to the shops. Once he started weaning he went back into a normal cycle.

Weaning started in early May when Dan was about eighteen weeks old.* Again he took to this quite quickly. We continued with breastfeeding alongside – but this then started to reduce to bedtime and early morning feeds. I returned to work when Daniel was five and a half months. When he was just short of seven months old he self-weaned completely from the breast – just decided one morning that he didn't want it, and the same for the next two or three mornings and the same at night. I think that particularly for the night-time feed I wasn't producing enough to keep him satiated.* I found this quite upsetting at the time as I wasn't ready to stop breastfeeding. David was very balanced about it and supported me through this.

We now have a healthy, lively, bright and cheeky four-year-old. Whilst we can't say that having breastfed Dan is a direct correlation to his health (although research does support it) – we have the contentment that we have given him the best start possible.

The benefits to the mother of immediate breastfeeding are innumerable, not the least of which after the weariness of labor and birth is the emotional gratification, the feeling of strength, the composure, and the sense of fulfillment that comes with the handling and suckling of the baby.

Ashley Montague

Sally's story

I always intended to breastfeed. My mum had breastfed us as children and I had grown up knowing that breast was best. I thought that I would try my best to do it, and if I couldn't manage it I wouldn't be too hard on myself. I had a close friend with three children who couldn't breastfeed so I was aware that it didn't always work out. When I look back now, though, I realise how devastating it would have been for me if we hadn't been successful.

I did what I could to prepare for breastfeeding. We attended NCT classes, and went to a session run by a breastfeeding counsellor at which they talked about technique. In retrospect, I'm not sure how much that helped: nothing can really prepare you for doing it yourself!

When Jasmine was born, I was lucky enough to have a pretty straightforward birth. I started having contractions in the morning, went to hospital at about 2pm, and Jasmine arrived at 9pm. I had gas and air, but no pethidine and no epidural. As soon as she was born, she had skin-to-skin with me and the midwife encouraged her to find the nipple, which she did and fed for around thirty minutes. We finally moved up to the ward from the delivery suite at about midnight and I was absolutely exhausted by then.

I clearly remember being woken up at about 3am – still completely shattered – by a lovely midwife who said it was time to feed my baby. I looked at her and just said "But I don't know how!". I was still so tired and in a daze that she practically did it for me, grabbing my boob and latching Jasmine on. In the morning, I dreamt that I hadn't fed her for ages – the night feed hadn't seemed real in my sleep-deprived state. I had to call the midwife again for help with feeding in the morning because I didn't feel at all confident. The hospital offered to discharge me that day, but I refused because I wanted to make sure I had absolutely nailed the feeding before I left. It really helped having Lyndon around when I was learning to feed because he seemed to be so good at listening to the advice they were giving me and helping me to do it. He could see the angle of Jasmine's head better than me as well, and he would hold her in position to latch her on.

All the feeds went well with someone to help me. I can't fault the midwives at the hospital (Derby Royal – a Baby-Friendly hospital); they were patient and helpful. They gave me the number of the infant feeding advisor who I could call if I had any problems, but I don't think I ever did.

Once we got home, there was a bit of a learning curve working out the best place to sit, which cushions to use and which position to feed in – I tended to prefer more upright sitting positions with a pillow on my lap. I can remember going to the first NCT coffee morning and wondering how on earth I would manage to feed Jasmine if she needed it, but we were all in the same boat and managed somehow. At home, we had visits from the community midwives and while they were all friendly and helpful, it was hard to build up a relationship with them because we saw a different one each time.

I didn't have many problems with breastfeeding – I can vaguely remember having some savoy cabbage leaves when I got a bit engorged, and I never knew whether to feed on one side or both, and how long for – and I could never remember which side I'd last fed on. In the end, we created some detailed charts to record which side I'd fed on and for how long, and at what time of day. I did try using a breastfeeding bracelet to remind me which side to feed on, but I was never sure whether I'd remembered to switch it over from the last time!

The only negative thing that I can remember is that my health visitor was pretty unhelpful and seemed to think Jasmine was underweight, despite the fact that she was clearly thriving. I knew that the charts she was using were not the ones that should be used for breastfed babies, so every time she mentioned weight I would get irritated and tell her that Jasmine's weight was fine on the breastfed baby charts from the WHO (World Health Organisation). The health visitor also suggested formula top-ups quite early on, but I had no confidence in her advice and did my own thing. She also mentioned moving to solids a lot earlier than I planned and again I ignored her. I felt then (and still do) that poor advice from health visitors does not help new mums to breastfeed and make the best informed decisions about how to feed and wean their children.

I didn't read many books that dealt with breastfeeding. I got most of my tips from a friend who has five children and an amazing memory for what she did with each child when they were small. It was she who suggested that we try Jasmine on a four-hour routine, feeding at 2pm, 6pm, 10pm, 2am, 6am and 10am. This seemed to suit Jasmine really well and she started to sleep better. The night wakings had been difficult and at times, when I was awake, alone, feeding Jasmine in the middle of the night I would look over at Lyndon, fast asleep, and feel quite lonely and as if I was experiencing parenthood differently from him.

We'd been given all the bottle-feeding paraphernalia – steriliser, bottles and a hand breast pump. I tried to express but found it quite an effort with the hand pump and didn't get much out. I went out to a hen party when Jasmine was a couple of months old and Lyndon tried to give her a bottle of expressed milk while I was out – she wasn't keen at first but eventually took it. When she was three months old, we left her for a whole day for the first time.

I'd been expressing like mad to get together enough breastmilk for her to last the whole day, and had been frustrated at the small amounts I would get. To add insult to injury, when I expressed while we were away that day I got more milk than ever before: it was literally gushing out. And we had to throw it away, having no means of storing it and taking it home. It was soul-destroying to see precious breastmilk thrown out of the car window into the bushes. I can still remember that feeling very clearly.

When Jasmine was born, we were a bit worried about how we would manage to get out and about, particularly as we had a host of important events to attend (weddings, a seventieth birthday party and so on), and the first of these was when Jasmine would be only six weeks old. We feared that, being new to parenthood, everyone would descend on us and think they knew how best to care for our baby. This was one of the reasons why we discouraged overnight visitors for the first couple of weeks that we were at home with Jasmine – we felt we had to get to know her on her own first. This set us up well for our hectic social calendar, and after the first event we knew what we had to do: fling everything in the car, feed to the schedule, and hope for the best! The good thing about needing to get out and about early on was that we soon got used to it and Jasmine took it all in her stride. We found it easy to take her to France when she was six months old, and we took her on a flight. I fed her on take off and landing to help her ears equalise. I found the special breastfeeding tops helpful for feeding in public. Before I had Jasmine, I had thought they would be a waste of money and was determined not to buy any, but I changed my mind once I realised how practical they were.

We started weaning when Jasmine was six months old and she seemed to enjoy her puréed veg and took to it well. I was still feeding her five times a day at first. By the time she went to nursery at seven months, I was feeding her before and after nursery and at night. She would have had formula – if she would have let it pass her lips! She didn't seem to like the taste and we worried about it, but she was eating well and having breastfeeds at home, so for a while she didn't have much milk at nursery.

Jasmine self-weaned when she was nine and half months old. By then she was only feeding in the evenings, and one night she just turned away. I wasn't ready to give up and it did feel like a rejection. I felt quite sad that we had finished breastfeeding, as I knew that Jasmine would be the only baby I breastfed, but on the other hand there was a sense that one chapter had ended and a new one had begun. I also felt a sense of satisfaction that she had chosen to stop of her own accord.

The downside of Jasmine self-weaning before a year old was that it left us the problem of what milk to give her until she could go on to cow's milk at a year. We tried various formulas with little success, until one day we picked up a carton of ready-mixed formula that she seemed to like. She had this in a bottle and then we had another round of weaning her off the bottle/formula and onto cow's milk/beakers!

Overall, I found breastfeeding an overwhelmingly positive experience. Once I became confident feeding in public, which happened quite early on, I just got on with it and never experienced any negativity. I used to go out to a nice restaurant with a couple of friends with breastfeeding babies and we would all quite happily "get them out" and feed. I'm not sure what the other diners thought but they never said anything! We did have good support from our families: my mum would have been horrified if I hadn't breastfed Jasmine, and although I could tell Lyndon's dad didn't really like me feeding in front of him, generally we felt that our families totally approved of what we were doing.

I'm going to do it as long as I can. There is something so intimate about it. For that one hour or forty-five minutes it's just wonderful. It's wonderful bonding and you know they're getting all those antibodies.

Catherine Zeta Jones

A baby nursing at a mother's breast... is an undeniable affirmation of our rootedness in nature.

David Suzuki

Joanna's story

I always knew I'd breastfeed. Apart from all the 'best for baby' advice it just seemed like the most natural thing to do. Throughout my pregnancy I'd been amazed at my body's ability to expand and nurture the new life inside me so I thought I'd trust it to feed the baby too. It wasn't until I went to an NCT workshop on breastfeeding as part of our antenatal classes that I realised it might not be so easy and came away with lots of potential problems, including the scary fact that a very small number of women do not produce milk. We were shown just one method of how to latch a baby on to the breast – the 'baby led' way. This is where the mother reclines and supports her baby as he finds his own way on to the nipple. In hindsight this four-hour workshop would have been much better if we were shown more methods of how to latch a baby to the breast. The thought of not being able to breastfeed compelled me to do enough research to be able to send my husband Dan out to buy bottles/pumps and all the other paraphernalia we might need if we had a problem but, feeling positive, we didn't buy any formula or equipment before the birth.

The birth itself was a wonderful, straightforward experience. My waters broke at 9.45pm and Ellen emerged at 3am the following day in an empty birthing pool in our kitchen. The midwife didn't arrive until 1am, by which point I was fully dilated and there was no time to start filling the pool! I remember Ellen coming out in one big contraction and being placed straight on my chest, half wrapped in a towel. She was incredibly slippy, screaming and still curled up like she had been in the womb. It was a little tricky to hold her and position her to suckle while trying to keep her warm and not let the towel fall off. I managed it but only with my husband Dan's finger pushing my breast away from Ellen's nose so she could breathe as she fed.

After about ten minutes Ellen was passed out of the pool to be weighed and dressed. Dan held her while I had a few stitches (which were by far the worst part of the birthing experience). By the time I'd been mended and got out of the pool Ellen was fast asleep in her moses basket. We all went upstairs, I had a shower and we were in bed by 6am and got a couple of hours sleep.

When we awoke I fed Ellen sitting up in bed. I didn't even attempt the 'baby led' way as she seemed too small and weak to nuzzle around and find a nipple. So with a bit of patience we learnt together – and finding a good position came naturally.

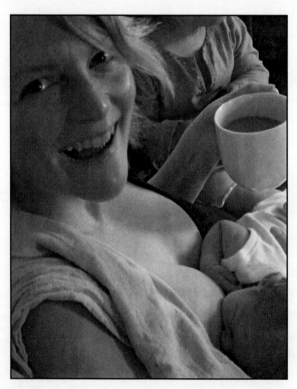

But I am glad I didn't have any 'help' from a midwife because it felt like one of those new skills that are best learnt in peace without anyone watching. However, I had no idea how to get Ellen to unlatch and in the middle of the night I would be so tired but unable to release my nipple from a sleepy Ellen. It was the midwife on day three who told me how I must break the seal around Ellen's mouth by inserting a finger in between her gums next to my nipple.

One thing I wasn't prepared for was the two seconds of pinching pain each time Ellen latched on. It disappeared after a few weeks, thankfully. Neither was I prepared for having a massive appetite. I thought I was hungry throughout pregnancy, but this was something else – two breakfasts, mid-morning, mid-afternoon and evening snacks, on top of lunch and dinner! And I really craved sweet things. Thirst was also a feature in my feeding routine and a glass of water was an essential. I'd often sit down without it though. That's where Dan was so supportive, getting up at 6am to make toast and fetching glasses of water on a regular basis.

I thought my milk had come in on day three as my breasts seemed huge and I had plenty of milk – but I woke on day four feeling like my breasts had turned into hot boulders. They were massive! The nursing bras I had been measured for at thirty-seven weeks would not do the job and I wasn't up to a shopping trip, so Dan received instruction with the help of the internet on bra measuring. I was thrilled to discover that I was now a whopping 36DD compared with my tiny 32A pre-pregnancy state. It must be mother nature's way of making up for the fact that you have a deflated football for a belly; she balances it out with a rack that a Page Three model would be proud of! I did enjoy having a good pose in the mirror. That said they were tender, leaking milk and not sexy. And that was a strange feeling in itself, to have the biggest breasts of my life and them not be sexual. Once again my body had transformed and I had another level of respect for it.

Along with the arrival of my milk I also experienced a new heightened feeling of emotion – good things like opening birth congratulation cards were wonderful and filled me with an indescribable amount of love and happiness for the world. But sad news on the radio would have me in floods of tears in seconds. I don't think I've fully recovered from it either!

Fortunately Ellen fed well and the heat and tenderness went down. From there on I didn't have any problems getting Ellen latched on or with her weight gain. The little weight she'd lost shortly after birth went back on quickly and the midwife checks passed without incident.

As my strength returned and I started to get out and about my next challenge was feeding in public (I didn't count feeding in front of family and visiting friends as public). My first attempt happened by chance when I was out for a walk and I fed on a bench in the park – Dan happened to be there which was good, because you do feel a bit vulnerable settling down to feed knowing that you can't make any quick movements. We got a lot of pleasant interest from a couple of middle-aged women who passed by – I think the sight of a suckling baby filled them with a sense of nostalgia. No one else in the park either noticed or cared. From there I graduated to feeding in a café with my NCT group, which was easy enough once I'd thought about which tops allowed easy access and learnt the art of using a muslin to cover up with. I also learnt the importance of wearing breast pads to deal with the inevitable leaking, which are easy to forget but not once you've had the experience of making DIY ones out of tissue in a café toilet!

The trouble with feeding in public began at about three months when Ellen was easily distracted and strong enough to pop herself off. So she would pull herself away from my breast, usually with a yell, taking the muslin with her, leaving me exposed, leaking milk, and soaking both me and her! This did make me feel a bit more anxious about being in public, especially if she didn't latch on straight away, which is more likely to happen in an unfamiliar place with lots of distractions for her. Still, I've only had one negative reaction. That came from a woman in a café, who upon realising I was about to feed a hungry, unhappy baby, loudly asked her husband if he wanted to swap seats so he wouldn't be in full view! I was a bit shocked that the sight of a lactating woman could cause such offence – especially as only someone paying careful attention would even realise a baby was being fed. As it turned out Ellen wouldn't settle down to feed so we left the café pronto. I wonder if she'd picked up the negative vibes from the neighbouring table – or maybe she'd sensed that I was tense.

At around ten weeks I thought it would be useful if Ellen could be fed from a bottle, the idea being that I could leave expressed milk for her and go off for a couple of hours. There was no great imperative for someone other than me to feed Ellen – I wasn't going back to work for a year – but I liked the idea of having the flexibility. And I took on board a comment a friend made about the 'danger of losing your sense of self' if I didn't have time away from the baby.

So after buying all the kit, reading the instructions and sterilising it all, at a time when I had enough milk and the time to express it – I managed to get about 100ml in about twenty minutes. I didn't enjoy the experience, I felt a bit like a cow! When it came to bottle-feeding time Ellen wouldn't take it, even from Dan when I was in another room. We tried about three more times and unfortunately neither Dan nor Ellen had any fun or success with it. I felt a little frustrated, until I realised that the six-month weaning mark would come around very quickly, and given that we don't live near family who could be regular babysitters it was unlikely that I would suddenly gain a huge amount of freedom anyway. After that I relaxed about the bottle-feeding, we went on holiday (without taking the equipment) and I didn't express any more milk. As for my sense of self, I think that's changed so much just from becoming a mother – but I don't think I'm in any grave danger of it disappearing!

On the whole I've found breastfeeding easy and I enjoy it immensely; it is fabulous to feel that my body is continuing to nurture our baby. At the time of writing Ellen is fifteen weeks old and I'm hoping to continue breastfeeding up until weaning at twenty-six weeks and beyond – whether or not she takes a bottle before then is still open to question.

Verity's story

I always assumed I would breastfeed my children: I am one of four siblings – myself and my sister Aby are identical twins, and we have an older sister and a younger brother – and my mother breastfed us all, so I never really considered bottle-feeding as an option.

When I was pregnant with my first son, I had quite severe oedema of the breasts; that is, they were swollen and the nipples became almost flat. I didn't realise the impact this might have on breastfeeding, and put it down to being one of those minor pregnancy complaints. I don't think I even mentioned it to my midwife.

I had Gabriel in hospital in a normal delivery after being induced. I didn't have any pethidine but I did have an epidural. He had a very low heartbeat that recovered well and seemed fine at birth, so I tried to feed him straightaway but had difficulty getting him to latch on. My nipples were so flat he was slipping off them. Mum was there to encourage me, and the midwives tried to help a bit but I got the impression they were at a bit of a loss as to how to fix the problem. I don't think they had seen boobs like mine before! My twin sister Aby had recently had a baby and I knew that she was having most success feeding in the 'rugby ball' hold, so I tried that and it did seem a bit better.

I got a four-hour discharge – I was desperate to get home having planned a home birth in the first place – and once home we started to get concerned that Gabriel wasn't having enough wet nappies. Fortunately my community midwife was a breast-feeding specialist and she taught me to express my milk and syringe-feed Gabriel to 'make up' for his poor latch. My milk came in fine and I had some engorgement, which was relieved by the pumping. My midwife advised either looking at Gabriel, or at a picture of him, to help the milk flow when expressing.

It took two weeks of hard work to get breastfeeding properly established. The midwife came every day and every day we agreed a new plan to make sure Gabriel was getting enough. I had a log next to the bed of how much I'd fed, expressed and syringe-fed, which breast and for how long.

The strain of getting the feeding established while recovering from the birth and looking after my first baby took its toll emotionally. I resented the fact that I felt so on my own with the responsibility for the feeding and I felt real anger that Jim, my husband, couldn't really help and would be asleep in another room while I was up in the night struggling. I didn't realise it at the time but this was the beginning of post-natal depression (PND), which got worse as the weeks passed. I eventually gave up exclusive breastfeeding when Gabriel was three and a half months old, because my relationship with Jim was under such strain and it felt as if sharing the feeding might help in some way. I combine-fed for about a month and then went over to formula completely.

Ironically the PND got a lot worse once I'd stopped breastfeeding, no doubt due to the hormonal changes that took place. I did get treated and started anti-depressants which really helped, and at the time I felt slightly relieved that I didn't have to consider the safety of taking the tablets while breastfeeding, although I now know that there are anti-depressants that are compatible with continuing to feed.

I did feel positive about the fact that I had got breastfeeding established despite the problems with oedema, but on the whole the experience hadn't worked out as I'd expected.

By the time I had my second son, Rupert, I was determined to breastfeed for longer, partly because I now knew about the protective effects of breastfeeding on PND. With Rupert I decided to have an independent midwife from the start, in the hope of ensuring that the whole birth experience would be closer to how I felt it should be. One great thing about this was that my midwife had the time to research breast oedema, and she discovered that there were ways to combat the problem. She accompanied me to a GP appointment at which we managed to get a referral to a specialist in breast oedema who ran a clinic in Nottingham. Most of the women seen by the specialist had breast cancer, and he had never seen oedema in pregnancy before, but having examined me he agreed that the manual lymphatic drainage massage he used with his other patients would work for me, and compression bras might also be helpful.

I had a wonderful home water birth with Rupert and I found it much easier to establish breastfeeding second time round. I did find my log useful again to remind me which breast he had fed from – in fact he developed a marked preference for one breast, to the extent that by five months I was feeding him exclusively on his preferred side and my supply adapted to that. I had intended to feed Rupert for at least a year to eighteen months, or even to let him naturally wean himself, but at seven and a half months he started biting me frequently during feeds. Despite my best efforts to distract him from this he persisted and in the end we moved over to bottles – so he effectively self-weaned, although a lot earlier than I would have liked.

I didn't suffer from PND after Rupert's birth, and found that many of the anxieties I'd had with Gabriel were no longer a concern. My relationship with Jim was much better and he was more involved with the birth and the early days. I co-slept with Rupert and in all our life was much more baby-focussed, which made us all feel more relaxed.

I felt that I had really benefited from the massage, the compression bras and the experience and care of my independent midwife. I had more antenatal appointments than I had with Gabriel, and they were longer (over an hour) each time, with plenty of time for talking. It was almost like therapy and I think helped the whole experience seem calmer and smoother.

My next pregnancy was with twins and I intended to breast-feed them from the outset. My sister had given birth to twins and had had some oedema problems that might have contributed to problems she had with breastfeeding them, so I was wary and ensured I was referred to the specialist lymph oedema clinic early on to get the compression bras fitted. They were interested to monitor my case and took photographs for a study they were working on. I now think that the problem is likely to be more common in pregnancy than is currently thought, as I suspect that many women, like me, think it is a minor inconvenience of pregnancy and not a treatable condition that can have knock-on effects on the success of breastfeeding.

With the twins I had set aside four full weeks to establish breast-feeding and I arranged support from family and friends to enable me to concentrate on the feeding. I spent a lot of time in bed with the twins and had lots of support from my independent midwife. The twins' birth had been eventful: twin one born in a rapid home birth, twin two born by caesarean after a transfer for placental abruption. I was glad to have all the hormones from the home birth doing their job as I tried to get the girls latched on! One twin got the hang of it straight away while the other took a while to get going – in the meantime I collected milk from the other breast in a breast shell while feeding and gave it to her by syringe.

Fortunately all went well and by two to three weeks, despite the usual odd wobble about weight gain and whether it was all working as well as I thought, breastfeeding the twins was well established. I used my logs again to plan and felt more confident about setting my own targets.

I co-fed the twins (that is, both at the same time, each on 'her' breast, in the rugby ball hold) because that was how Mum had fed us. Other holds didn't feel as comfortable. Right from the start I would try to feed them together, and would wake the other when one woke for a feed. I felt that this helped keep their routines on an even keel. Contrary to the myth, breastfeeding didn't stop my girls from sleeping well – by five to six months they were regularly sleeping through.

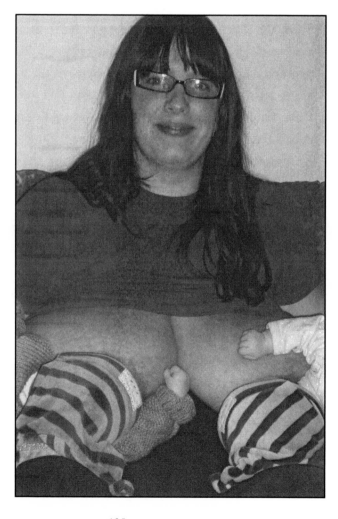

After a couple of months I did get some soreness and cracked nipples, I think just due to the increased wear and tear of having twins feeding frequently. I also had a bout of mastitis. I recognised it for what it was early on and got the antibiotics needed to treat it, but they stripped out my gut and I then got very ill with a diarrhoea and vomiting virus. I was ill for four weeks and managed to breastfeed through it, although I was quite taken aback when Jim and my Mum, normally so supportive of breastfeeding, urged me to give it up to give myself time to recover from the illness. I felt very strongly that I wanted to continue and would have felt cheated if I had allowed the illness to force an early end to breastfeeding, so I persevered.

At eight and half months the twins still get virtually all of their fluids from me. I give them the odd cup of water with meals but I am very proud to still be providing all of their milk.

With the twins I had suffered from antenatal depression, and was referred to the perinatal psychiatric unit. Although I had reservations about attending, it was very helpful and we devised an action plan to deal with any PND that might develop after the birth. I was prescribed a prophylactic dose of an anti-depressant compatible with breastfeeding to start immediately after the birth. On the day I wasn't sure if I would begin taking them, but I did. There are long-term studies that point to the safety of these drugs, and I was told that the benefits to the girls of breastfeeding would outweigh the very small risk of side-effects from the anti-depressants.

Breastfeeding the twins has been an immensely empowering experience. At first I wasn't sure if I would feed them in public, but my midwife firmly told me that it was a feminist issue and that I absolutely should be doing my bit to normalise breastfeeding and women's capabilities by getting on with feeding while out and about. So I did, and I have had nothing but positive feedback and never had a negative comment.

While I have been feeding the twins my older boys have been very interested in the whole process, to the extent that they seemed keen to try the milk. One night I expressed some while in the bath and gave it to them in a cup to taste. They didn't like it!

Overall breastfeeding my children has been immensely important to me. I think what I have learned is that the way our society deals with breastfeeding means that women often need huge amounts of support to be successful, because we don't have the kind of communal knowledge we need from mothers, grandmothers and sisters. We rely on the professionals and the volunteers to help us and it can be hard to access that level of support, especially in the newborn period when you have so much to deal with anyway.

Mother's milk, time-tested for millions of years, is the best nutrient for babies because it is nature's perfect food.

Robert S. Mendelsohn

A newborn baby has only three demands. They are warmth in the arms of its mother, food from her breasts, and security in the knowledge of her presence. Breastfeeding satisfies all three.

Grantly Dick-Read

Laura's story

I never really had any strong feelings on breastfeeding before I had my daughter; no one in my family had breastfed and I knew very little about what to expect. My midwife covered it in my antenatal class but I was more concerned about giving birth than what was to come after! However, breastfeeding was what was recommended so I was going to give it a go.

When my baby eventually arrived it was a bit of a shock to say the least. After an easy labour and water birth Madelyn Amy Phillips was born on 1 July 2006 weighing 7lb 3oz. I put Maddy to the breast straight away and although I was unprepared she seemed to know exactly what she wanted. Unfortunately, despite an easy labour I had a nasty tear and was taken to theatre to be stitched up so me and my baby were separated. When she was given back to me one hour later, having cried the whole time I was away, I put her back on my breast, but the calm baby I had delivered seemed to be gone.

The next twenty-four hours were spent trying to latch her on properly. The midwives were very good and gave me lots of help, but it did involve some handling of my breast. Madelyn fed constantly and when visiting time arrived everyone came at the same time. When I look back on it now I realise how daunting that must have been, trying to feed with six people all sat looking at me. On my second night in hospital the nurses took Maddy away for a while so I could get a little sleep.

By the time I got home my nipples were cracked and bleeding but I was doing well. By day three my hormones had well and truly caught up with me, as had the lack of sleep, and I became very tearful. The constant round of visitors didn't help. My stitches were painful, my baby wouldn't stop crying, I was exhausted and it felt like everyone was watching me. I was starting to feel like a freak show. My husband Darren tried to help as much as he could, but every time I closed my eyes he would appear with a crying baby who constantly wanted my breast. Maddy suffered with wind and the only way to relieve it was to feed her, but then she'd be sick. I couldn't understand why she was feeding so much and a lot of it was comfort feeding. What was I doing wrong?

By week three I was still crying all the time and I was getting a lot of conflicting advice from midwives, health visitors and others. A lot of people were starting to tell me to give it up and put Maddy on the bottle. I didn't know what I wanted and it started to feel inevitable as I had little success with expressing. I reached rock bottom in week four when Darren returned to work, my mum was on holiday and I'd had three hours sleep. I

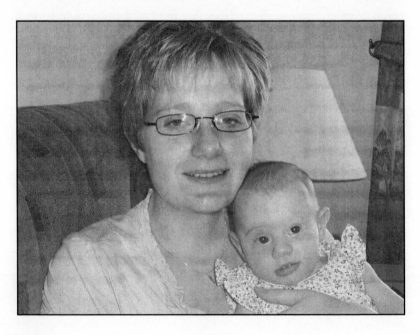

felt so alone that as I sat with my baby in my arms and we both cried I uttered the words "What have I done?".

Having reached my lowest point it was then that I went to BIBS, a local breastfeeding group, in the hope they could tell me what I was doing wrong, but it turned out I wasn't doing anything wrong. Newborn babies are meant to feed a lot and when someone said that "As long as she was on my breast the tigers wouldn't get her" it somehow made sense to me. At that group for the first time someone told me I was doing well. I'd breastfed my baby for four weeks.

After a couple of weeks of going to BIBS and giving Maddy something for her wind, the weather started to cool down and I had turned a corner. By the time she was six weeks old I was feeling much better and decided to carry on.

From then on I started to enjoy breastfeeding. Some of my happiest memories with Maddy are of her feeding, although it was a long time before I got a full night's sleep, nine months to be exact. I didn't mind. My baby and I would curl up under a blanket in her nursery while everyone else slept: in fact, this is how we saw in Madelyn's first new year. I don't know if breastfeeding has any effect on the mother's immune system, but I felt great.

I may have had my ups and downs, but meeting other mums who were going through the same as me helped me to gain confidence.When Madelyn was nine months old I became a peer supporter for Bills, another local breastfeeding group.

I finally stopped breastfeeding when Maddy was fourteen months, after a gradual process of cutting down. It doesn't matter when I stopped feeding, but it's important that I stopped when the time was right for me and not when other people thought I should.

*****

If there's one thing that didn't worry me about having another baby it was breastfeeding. In fact, it's what I was looking forward to most. Maddy was two and a half when I fell pregnant and after what can only be described as the world's worst pregnancy I gave birth on 20 October 2009.

I had an elective C-section due to my previous tear. Although people told me breastfeeding would be extremely difficult, I was pretty confident. I spoke to the breastfeeding counsellor at Bills about what the challenges would be and she confirmed what I already knew: my milk would come in late and positioning could be tricky. One thing I did know was how important skin-to-skin was.

Maisie was born weighing 7lb ¾oz and when I was back in recovery following my C-section I put her skin-to-skin for her first feed. Fortunately both me and baby were well and just like her sister she knew exactly what to do. I followed her lead and allowed her to latch on herself. Most of her feeds I did this way. I found self-attachment so much easier and as she was my second baby I was pretty much left to get on with it.

The first night after she was born she fed loads but I knew this was normal and I only had a tiny amount of soreness and bleeding from my nipples. Practically every feed I did skin-to-skin. I'm sure people thought I was off my rocker stripping my baby off every time I fed her. But I was doing well, and Maisie seemed to be a very chilled baby and slept loads.

On day three I was all set to take my baby home, but the nurse weighed her and discovered that she had lost more than ten per cent of her body weight. This was when it was suggested that I give her some formula. Don't get me wrong, if my baby had been becoming poorly, I would have given her formula, but her glucose levels were ok and this was really not what I wanted so I told the nurse.

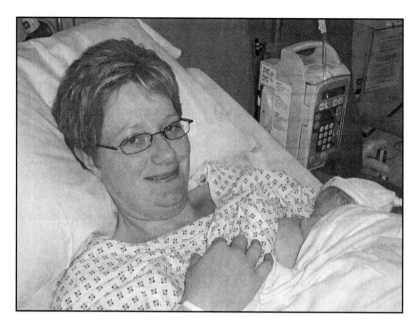

The paediatrician asked me to express to give us an idea of how much I was producing.* This reassured everyone that I was producing a good amount of milk; in fact I was expressing when my milk came in. Thankfully my wishes were respected and the paediatrician agreed that as I was feeding her myself I should continue, but wake her every three hours to feed.

I made it home the following day and unlike when Maddy came home from hospital it was wet and cold. I will always remember this day as one of my most favourite moments. Darren had cleaned the house, we put a ban on visitors and I could hear Madelyn laughing upstairs as she played with Daddy, while I cuddled up on the settee feeding my beautiful new baby, watching *Father of the Bride part two* and waiting for pizza to be delivered. Happy days!

Having to wake Maisie during the night was not easy. If she wanted to feed she would but if she wanted sleep... Thankfully her weight gain had improved and the midwife agreed I should go back to feeding on demand.

These early days with Maisie were not as difficult as when I had Maddy. The visitors aren't as constant second time round and I was so much more confident. Maddy took to her little sister very well and although it was a long time before I could get into any kind of a routine, and I had my moments of tearfulness, I managed to keep it together.

It was around week four that I contracted mastitis. I had noticed that one side of my breast was sore and when I began to get the flu-like symptoms that come with it I knew exactly what I was dealing with. I contacted the doctor and he gave me antibiotics, but I knew the only way to really get rid of it was to feed, so I changed position and within a couple of days I could feel the blockage flush away.

As I write this Maisie is ten months old and thriving. As I look back over the last ten months I realise I have been so much more relaxed about feeding and had I not had the confidence to follow

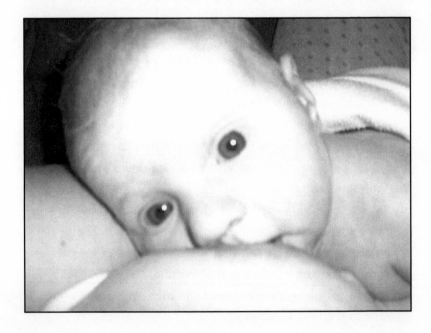

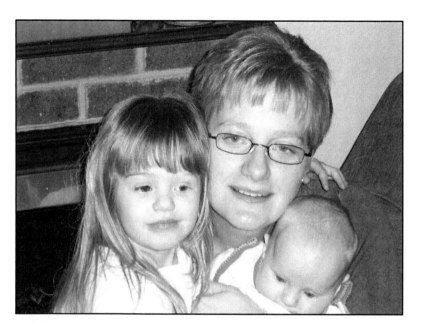

my instincts when I was in hospital, this could have been a very different story. Despite the ups and downs I have enjoyed every minute. I don't know when I will stop feeding and as Maisie is my last baby it will be with great sadness that I stop. But I will always be glad that I persevered and gave my girls the very best start in life.

While breastfeeding may not seem the right choice for every parent, it is the best choice for every baby.

Amy Spangler

All I ever heard was everyone bitch about it, nobody ever said, 'You are not going to believe how emotional this is.'

Jennifer Garner

Claire's story

I'd always intended to breastfeed, even before I went to ante-natal classes and learned more about the benefits for me and the baby. My mum hadn't breastfed my brother and me – it was the 1970s, and she was fully bought in to the "formula milk is amazing" idea – but for me the health benefits for the baby were paramount and the main reason that I thought breastfeeding was important. My husband Rob thinks that I thought breastfeeding would be easier – less hassle than all the sterilising and making up bottles – but I don't think that was a factor in my decision that it was the right thing to do. While I was pregnant one of my midwives told me at an antenatal appointment that giving even one bottle of formula can knock out some of the benefits of breastfeeding – even if this was not strictly accurate it did reinforce my commitment to do my best to feed exclusively for six months as the guidelines suggest.

When Jessica was born I had a fairly quick and straightforward natural delivery – with no time for any pain relief because we'd only been in the delivery suite for half an hour! We tried latching her on straight away, but she was jaundiced and sleepy and didn't feed well then. I'd had Jess at 10.30pm and we stayed in hospital that night and the following night to try to get the feeding sorted out. An unhelpful midwife with a stroppy bedside manner woke me up in the night and ordered me to wake Jess up and feed her – I was feeling exhausted and her approach left me feeling tearful and miserable as Jess wouldn't wake properly and feed. I cried about it to another midwife who was more proactive and actually hand-expressed some colostrum for me, so that I could finger-feed it to Jess and I would know that she was getting something. This did help, even if all my dignity had gone out of the window! I soon realised that in some ways you do end up giving up your rights to your body while you are feeding.

It took me about six weeks to feel that we'd got breastfeeding properly established. Just as things seemed easier, Jess had an accident that caused an injury to her mouth that swelled and really set the breastfeeding back. It was painful for her to latch on and her gum and lip were swollen. We took her to hospital and she was kept in overnight. While we were in hospital she wouldn't latch on, and while we were waiting around I became very engorged and she was hungry. I asked for a breast pump so that I could express milk for her. Overnight she was tube-fed my expressed milk. For a while afterwards she had to be fed expressed milk by syringe. I had to keep expressing at home to keep up my supply, and Jess did have some expressed milk by bottle as well – at that age she took bottles fairly well, but later on, when we wanted her to have bottles at around six months, she was much less accommodating and I eventually had to go out for a very long walk, leaving her with Rob, until the bottle was drunk and he rang to say I could come home!

The accident and injury to Jess's face left me feeling very cross – although I knew it was an accident it had set us back a long way when I had struggled to get the feeding sorted out in the first place. However, the whole incident really underlined my commitment to breastfeeding – it would have been so easy, when Jess was taken into hospital, to think that formula might have been easier than the expressing and syringe-feeding, but it wasn't what I wanted for her so I persevered with the breastfeeding.

While we were getting feeding established I had a cracked nipple, which is a common complaint and often down to a slightly wonky latch. I told my health visitor about it and she wrote it in my red book and advised me to attend a local breastfeeding group. I thought about phoning one of the breastfeeding helplines but didn't do so – I couldn't see how they could help me without seeing the problem. It seemed like too much effort, as a first-time mum, to attend a group – I wasn't sure I liked the idea of my problems being chewed over in a group setting – so I didn't go. Another midwife or maternity assistant suggested trying the rugby ball hold to change the latch a little, but I found that didn't come naturally and didn't help.

The wife of one of Rob's work colleagues, whom I didn't know well, had a baby about five months before Jess was born. When Jess arrived she sent us some bits and bobs and a lovely letter advising me to try Lansinoh nipple cream and to buy Clare Byam-Cook's book *What to Expect When You're Breastfeeding...And What If You Can't?** I followed her advice and in the end the cracked nipple cleared up and feeding was no longer painful. It was lovely of this lady who hardly knew me to give me the benefit of her experience to help keep me going – she obviously knew that breastfeeding could be tough. I hope this book is going to do the same sort of thing for other women.

Overall I found that although there were some good health professionals (like the midwife in hospital who helped with the finger-feeding), I also came across plenty who were unapproachable. I really could have done with more active assistance with some of my breastfeeding problems, and I find it strange that the NHS is so keen to push the benefits of breastfeeding, without having proper support in place postnatally.

I found feeding in public quite awkward at first. I have quite large breasts and was worried about how much flesh was on display – not just the breasts, in fact, but the belly as well! I can remember the first time I fed in public was outside a café in a local park. I was with my NCT friends, which helped, but I still got flustered. I soon learned to be prepared, both by wearing breastfeeding-friendly clothing (vests, cardigans and so on) and by always having a muslin in my handbag to cover up any other bits.

When we went to Rob's parents' house I offered, in the beginning, to go into another room to feed the baby because they were obviously uncomfortable about my feeding in front of them. It was annoying because once I'd started doing this I didn't feel I could change it, even when I got more confident and realised I shouldn't have to hide away and feel isolated from the family. By the time I had Lucy (my second daughter, born when Jess was two) I was much more confident and felt it was important to stand up for myself, so I don't go into another room any more.

I bought a feeding poncho when I had Jess, mainly because we were going to visit a friend who was 'funny' about breastfeeding and who had a thirteen-year-old son whom we had thought might be a bit embarrassed about my feeding. However, the poncho was useless and made me much more conspicuous than if I had just got on with it in the normal way. I'm now selling it on Ebay! Tops with scarves have been more useful for feeding discreetly.

I'd always intended to feed Jess exclusively for six months, and a couple of months after that I had a big hen weekend to attend which felt like a bit of a deadline. So when we got to six months I began to drop a feed a week, replacing it with formula, and we were all done with breastfeeding by the time Jess was eight months. I felt ready to move on, and more than ready to get rid of the hideous feeding bras. I burnt one ceremonially in a cheminea at my brother's house – declaring that was it, I wouldn't be needing it any more. Ironically, on the way home we got stuck in awful traffic and didn't have any bottles with us, so I ended up doing a last feed or two that I hadn't planned on, which was funny after my grand giving-up gesture!

When Lucy was born I knew I would breastfeed her too. I had her at home, hoping to avoid some of the hospital experiences I'd had first time around, and I was lucky enough to have a lovely midwife at my birth, with vast amounts of experience, who checked my latch and made sure Lucy was on well. I was also much more confident that I knew what I was doing. Having said that, it still hurt at first and I did experience some cracking of the nipples – but I now realise that each time Mum and baby need to learn how to feed from scratch, it's a skill that you have to practice and get right. Experience definitely helps, though, and within two weeks it felt as though we'd got the feeding properly established, much more quickly than I had with Jess. I can feed her in the dark, at night, because she latches on so well herself (she's now nearly twelve weeks).

Second time around I was delighted to discover that I didn't have to have the same awful nursing bras I'd had for Jess. Those had come from the NCT bra adviser, but they didn't suit my shape or offer me enough support, and were expensive. You might think that the type of bra you wear for feeding doesn't really matter, but it can affect your self-esteem, and let's face it, you're going to be wearing them a lot. With Lucy I found a great shop in Nottingham that sold Hot Milk bras – beautiful, supportive and a really worthwhile investment.

I have found it challenging feeding a newborn while caring for my toddler – Jess has watched a lot of Peppa Pig lately! But I can't see how bottles and formula would make that any easier, and I can't imagine not doing the same for Lucy as I did for Jess in terms of giving her the best start. I was surprised and a bit shocked when I overheard some other mothers saying that they regretted breastfeeding their second children because it had been such a hassle. It can be difficult but I am sure it is worth it.

When Lucy was a few weeks old we took Jess to Drayton Manor, a theme park for children. I had checked their website beforehand and was pleased to see that they had breastfeeding facilities. However, when we got there I asked a member of staff and was directed to a room next to the toilets, which was not much better than an actual toilet itself. It had one hard chair and an overflowing nappy bin that smelled awful – no one would want to feed a baby in there. I joined some other mothers who were sitting outside in the rain to feed rather than use the 'facilities'. It makes me cross that so-called family-friendly attractions can get away with this kind of thing. They should take a leaf out of the Westfield Centre in Derby's book – there the parents' rooms are excellent, with comfy chairs, playpens for older children and good toilet and changing facilities.

I intend to feed Lucy for a similar length of time to Jess, but I'm keeping my options open. I know a bit more now about how I might be able to cut the feeds right down, but keep the night time or early morning ones, so I'll see how it goes. Overall, Rob and I both feel really positive about breastfeeding and are glad that I've managed to do it for both girls. At the moment it suits our family life very well – Rob works hard, has a long commute and I look after the girls during the week. If I had to add sterilising and making up feeds to my workload I think it would be difficult and I like the fact I don't have to think about feeding too much when planning my days. I do all the night feeds so that Rob can get a decent night's sleep, which can be hard but is the practical solution to the way our life is at the moment. It's a shame for Rob that he doesn't see much of the children during the week, and that I am tired out by them and by the feeding, and sometimes he does feel as if there's no time left in the day for just the two of us, but we can both see that time goes quickly and babies won't be tiny and breastfeeding forever. We feel strongly that it's been the right thing to do.

Kodi's story

NB: Kodi is in the US

There was never a question about whether or not I would breast-feed. It was a given. When I was pregnant with my first child, the only reason I registered for bottles was because I planned on holding on to my part-time job. I invested in a pump and gave the formula samples in my free "breastfeeding" diaper bag to the Salvation Army.

My mother breastfed my little sister for eighteen months. So that was my goal. When the teacher of the breastfeeding class at the hospital asked about goals, and I piped up with "eighteen months" after most said "six months", I received a few sidelong glances, but no criticism.

My first daughter was born on Thanksgiving weekend in 2003. My doctor was, of course, not the one on call, so I had a complete stranger in the room telling me I wasn't breathing! (Silly me, I was confused by all the oxygen going into my lungs!) I was in little pain until eight centimetres, and then opted for the epidural. During the purple pushing you have to do with an epidural, Dr Complete Stranger decided I was exhausted (without consulting me in the matter), and cut an almost fourth degree episiotomy because she was using the vacuum extractor.

"It's a girl!" was the first thing my husband said. Followed immediately by the exclamation, "She's beautiful!" I sat up as best I could and held out my arms for my baby. Dr Complete Stranger held her up so I could see her, then ignored my arms and passed her off to the nurses. She was swaddled and passed around to those in the waiting room before I got to see her again or hold her. I immediately offered her my breast. She licked at my nipple and put it in her mouth, but otherwise seemed too sleepy to do much else.

The next day or two at the hospital was a bit of a blur. She was sleepy and it took a while to get her to latch on, but after a while we managed it. As a first time mom, I was unsure if she was latched on correctly, but every time the lactation consultation was there, all she did was sleep.

Her paediatrician advised me to time her feedings. So many minutes on one breast, then switch, gradually upping the amount of minutes on a breast. He made it seem so complicated! And the nurses were constantly calling me, asking how many minutes she nursed and how many diapers. Whoever says a new mom gets rest after birth in a hospital, didn't go to that one!

We brought our precious angel home and our lives changed for the better. That was her nickname, Angel. My milk came in a few days later and my breasts were hard as a rock! They hurt and they were so high up on my chest they were practically under my chin. I had to hand express a bit of milk just so she could latch on. And once she got the milk flowing, there was no holding it back. She gulped and sputtered and coughed and drank as fast as she could to keep from drowning! (I had a fast letdown, but didn't know it: more on that later.)

As a result she spit up quite a bit. My mom even remarked, "I thought breastfed babies didn't spit up?" But it didn't seem to bother her any, so I thought nothing of it.

She developed a touch of jaundice. The doctor advised me to give her sugar water with a syringe to flush it out. We tried once to give it to her and it was a complete disaster. She wanted no part of that stuff! So we threw it out and I just nursed her. Nursing flushed the jaundice out and she was fine.

Although she had a bit of a slow start, once she figured out the nursing thing, she could not get enough! She nursed every forty-five minutes to an hour, almost around the clock. All the books I had read beforehand had all said the same thing, breastfed babies nurse every two to three hours. Well, apparently Angel had not read the same books I had, so did not know how often she was supposed to eat! She quickly made me realise that all the books I had read were not going to be much help. I used one breast per feeding, and let her nurse on it until she decided she was done. It was so much easier than trying to keep track of minutes per breast and all the other things that made it so complicated. If it hadn't been that long between nursings, I just used the same breast.

I worked part-time as a school bus driver when she was born. I pumped a bottle for her in the morning. I went to work and was back before my husband had to go to work. Most of the time she slept the whole time I was gone. In the afternoons, a woman up the street watched her. When she was around five months old, school ended for the summer. After those wonderful days of spending all my time with her, I did not want to leave her again! So we decided I would not go back to work, and I became a stay at home mom.

When she was six months old we gave her a few bites of cereal and a bottle of diluted apple juice. Again, everything I read on feeding a baby was so complicated! After a few weeks of using a food grinder and trying to give her cereal (which smelled and tasted disgusting, no wonder she didn't like it) I threw up my hands and decided all the guidelines the experts were spouting were utter nonsense. From then on if I gave her any table food it was from my plate, mashed up or otherwise cut into tiny non-choking pieces. I paid no attention to whether she was getting veggies before fruits or anything else. I just fed her bites here and there of what I was eating.

She never ate much. She would go days without eating table foods. She was an expert nurser! I had no problems during the day, but at night the frequent nursing sessions were rough, even though we had her crib in our room. One night, after waking up five times in one hour to nurse her back to sleep, I thought "This is ridiculous!" and brought her to bed with me. She slept all night, and so did I! Sleeping with her cuddled up next to me was blissful. And the frequent night nursing barely affected our sleep as I was able to nurse her without either of us really waking up. We happily slept together from then on.

The closer we got to my goal of eighteen months the more I realized neither she nor I were ready to stop. There was no reason to stop, so we just continued. Both my husband and my mother were questioning when she was going to "stop that", but I just told them when we were ready to. I was surprised at my mother's disapproval, but it didn't change my mind. When my husband questioned it, I just told him some benefits to continued nursing and he would drop the subject. He had no real objection to it, just didn't know much about it. Besides, he wasn't doing the nursing, so I figured his vote was minimal!

*****

I become pregnant when Angel was nineteen months old. I researched nursing during pregnancy and concluded that, again, there was no reason to wean. After my experience in the hospital when Angel was born, I was keen to avoid a repeat of that, so I found a homebirth midwife to be my care provider. She was supportive of my continuing to nurse Angel.

The first trimester was a bit rough. Morning sickness has never been a friend to me, and it was no different this time around. Exhaustion and sore nipples made nursing Angel a bit hard to handle, but I honestly had no energy to try to wean even if I had decided to.

Around the end of the first trimester, I noticed it was taking longer and longer to nurse Angel to sleep. After taking a closer look, I realized I was no longer having a letdown. Soon after that, it was apparent that my milk was gone. Her frequent nursing sessions went down dramatically. She went from nursing five to eight times a day to twice! She did not like cow's milk, so she drank more juice than before.

Having no milk did not stop her from nursing. She still required nursing to go to sleep, but by then she was not taking naps, so it was just at nighttime. She still wanted to nurse during the day for comfort once or twice. Although latching on was a bit uncomfortable for me, nursing was easier then ever.

On my due date I awoke at 12.45 in the morning to visit the bathroom. My water broke while I was on the toilet! After a quick call to my midwife, I promised to call her when my contractions started. Contractions started about half an hour later. Because I had brought my midwife running for a false alarm a few weeks earlier, I waited until I was sure I was in labor before calling her. I waited a little too long! My midwife arrived at my house around 4.45am. I got in a hot shower soon after she arrived, and almost immediately felt ready to push! I got out of the shower and settled myself with a birthing stool in our bedroom. At 5.24am, our second daughter was born!

She latched on immediately as I cradled her close. She knew exactly what to do! When the cord stopped pulsing, it was cut as she nursed. She was awake and aware and her quick nursing helped deliver the placenta.

Angel was introduced to her new sister soon after, once I was settled into bed. Within an hour after birth I had both my girls nursing together, one on each breast.

*****

Tandem nursing took a bit of practice for us to get used to. I would latch the baby on first and then allow Angel to crawl up in my lap and nurse on the other side. In the evenings they would both fall asleep there and I would have my husband take Angel to bed.

Having learned my lesson with Angel, our new baby girl, nicknamed Little Bit, was brought right into bed with us from the first. Angel started out the night in a toddler bed in our room, but usually crawled into our bed sometime during the night. After a few nights of Angel wanting to nurse during the night more often than the newborn, I was exhausted! It was too much for me to handle, so I decided to night-wean Angel. I told her that she didn't nurse at night anymore, but that we would nurse when the sun came up. When she woke during the night asking to nurse, I offered her a cup of water or milk, and reminded her that we would nurse when the sun came up. She handled it very well. However there were several mornings when I woke up to her nursing! "Momma! Sun up!" She made sure I kept to my promise and nursed her upon waking.

Day nursing was easier now that I was only nursing one at night. I could rarely nurse Little Bit without Angel climbing up in my lap too. She reverted to newborn nursing, nursing frequently.

Little Bit also developed jaundice. Due to my success with Angel, I had no doubt we could nurse the jaundice away. My midwife also suggested sunbaths for her. We stripped her to a diaper and lay her in the sun a couple of times a day. The jaundice did not stay for long.

Little Bit had a different nursing schedule. She was a more average nurser, only needing to nurse every couple of hours. This completely baffled me and I had a hard time believing that she wasn't hungry even when it had only been an hour! Surely she was hungry and needed to nurse? It took me a while to listen to her cues and not worry that she didn't nurse as frequently as my first had.

Although she didn't nurse as often, other things were the same as in Angel's newborn days. Little Bit also coughed and sputtered and choked on my milk. I would have to nurse until the milk let down, and then pull her off and soak up the spray in a towel until it stopped. Then I would put her back on and let her finish. By this time we had gotten with the times and had internet access. I realized that I had a fast letdown with an oversupply. Just as I had with Angel. Block feeding (using one breast per feeding, or a specified amount of time) was a recommended technique. I had been doing that already, as I had success with Angel using that method. However, I had done it out of instinct.

The oversupply was not such a big problem this time around as I had a toddler! A toddler is a wonderful thing to have around when you are engorged. A toddler can get much more milk out than a newborn, so I had no issues with engorgement.

As Little Bit grew and thrived, Angel finally started reducing her frequent nursing sessions. A few months after Little Bit was born, Angel was no longer nursing to sleep. Then she decided she wanted to sleep in her own room. That was hard on me, as it was completely out of the blue and I was not prepared! But she was ready, and she did great.

I decided to take a more relaxed approach to solids this time. Little Bit was closer to eight months before we started giving her bites of our food. She ate whatever we ate.

Little Bit grew and thrived. Angel was down to a few nursings a day. When Little Bit was around eighteen months we sold our house and moved into a house in town. Nursing was a big constant during that time and was a big support in helping the girls settle into our new house. Little Bit slept in a toddler bed in our room (for some of the night) while Angel had her own room. We were all enjoying our new house.

I had an early miscarriage not long after we moved in. It hit me hard as I was excited about another baby. I only had a week or so of new baby joy before it was apparent that the pregnancy was not sustainable. My midwife helped me through it.

I was content with my two precious girls. They were my joy! Little Bit continued to nurse frequently during the day and night, while Angel was down to once, maybe twice.

Angel turned four years after we moved into our new house. The first time I mentioned that one day she would not nurse anymore, her eyes got really big and she looked shocked. It obviously hadn't occurred to her that she would have to stop nursing one day! We talked about it a few times to let her get used to the idea.

A couple of months after her fourth birthday, she started talking about how she was a big girl and big girls don't nurse. She would decide she didn't nurse anymore one afternoon and ask to nurse the next morning! The morning nursing was the only one she had left and she had a hard time letting that one go. After a while of her going back and forth, I finally had to refuse her one morning. I told her that she had decided she didn't nurse anymore, so I wasn't going to nurse her. After looking a little disappointed, she said ok. She was four years and five months old.

I was down to nursing one child. A couple of weeks later a voice in my head told me, "Kodi, you are pregnant." I told the voice it was wrong, that we were charting to prevent pregnancy. The voice continued to pop up in my head, saying those same four words. I took a pregnancy test just to prove that voice wrong. I was shocked to see a positive test.

A month after Angel weaned, I found myself pregnant!

*****

This pregnancy was a surprise. I was charting to prevent pregnancy. I can only assume that Angel weaning threw my cycle off and possibly caused me to ovulate twice. After the initial shock wore off I was cautiously ecstatic.

The first trimester was the same as the others. Sick, tired, nauseous and generally feeling rotten. The girls spent a lot of time watching television as I wallowed in misery on the couch. Again, nursing Little Bit was easy because it made her happy with the least amount of effort on my part.

By the end of the first trimester, I was feeling better. But it was obvious my milk was gone again. Little Bit continued to nurse, but she started asking for milk from the refrigerator. She drank a lot of cow's milk. We started going through three gallons of milk a week because she drank so much.

But she still needed to nurse to sleep. She still needed to nurse during the night. And she still needed to nurse during the day to help her when she got out of control. She would have a typical two-year-old temper tantrum and nursing calmed her down when nothing else would.

The girls were excited about having a new baby. For months they wanted it to be a boy, but by the end of the pregnancy they had changed their minds and wanted nothing else but a girl.

Little Bit would rub my growing belly as she nursed. Occasionally the baby would kick her as if to tell her "Quit crowding me!".

I went into labor on a Friday evening. Expecting a short labor as I had with Little Bit, and wanting to avoid my midwife getting there at the last minute, I called her around midnight. She got to our house around 4am. She told me to get some rest and I went to bed and got some sleep.

Labor continued all throughout the next day and evening. I was able to nurse Little Bit to sleep early in the evening, but when labor started revving up I was unable to nurse her back to sleep when she awoke. My husband's father was there and was able to take care of Little Bit. She was not happy and only fitfully dozed.

At 2am our third daughter was born. She was wet and warm and wonderful! She was too interested in looking at me to latch on right away. But after a little coaxing she finally decided to do it. Just like Little Bit she knew just what to do. Such a difference from my first daughter.

Little Bit was awake and met her new sister soon after. She was in awe and in love with her new sister! After all the excitement of birth, we nursed and snuggled down into bed and went to sleep, Little Bit, the new baby and me.

*****

Angel met her new sister the next morning. She was told of her new sister the night before, but told her father, "I'll see her in the morning Daddy." I guess she was too sleepy to get up in the middle of the night.

I was back to nursing a newborn and a toddler. I had been here before so I was able to use all the tips and tricks I had learned then, to help me now. Both Little Bit and the new baby, Sunshine, had no problems nursing together.

Little Bit was ecstatic that I had milk again! She stopped asking for milk from the refrigerator and went back to nursing full-time. She wanted to nurse every time the baby did. She would tell me "This nipple is for me and that one is for baby!" Although I never assigned sides, Little Bit was usually on my right and Sunshine was on my left most of the time.

I again had to night-wean. Little Bit was asking to nurse more often then the new baby and I couldn't handle that. So using the same method that worked with Angel, I night-weaned her. She was two years and eight months old.

I still had a fast flow and an oversupply. Sunshine would choke on my letdown. I kept a supply of towels close by to soak up the spray. After a few months she knew how to unlatch herself if the flow got too strong. But I still had to use the towels until she was around six months.

Sunshine grew and thrived. Little Bit continued her frequent nursing for months after Sunshine was born. I waited patiently (and sometimes not so patiently!) for her to decrease the nursings on her own. Finally it was almost a year before she finally stopped asking to nurse so often! If she had not started dropping nursing sessions on her own, I had already decided I was going to have to start limiting her.

When Sunshine was around eight months old she contracted an ear infection. Since this was my first time dealing with an ear infection, I panicked a little, and despite my knowledge that few ear infections require antibiotics, I filled the prescription the doctor gave me. The ear infection went away, but thrush took its place.

This was my first time dealing with thrush as well! The soreness was bad enough, but the burning when she nursed was worse. I treated her mouth and my nipple with gentian violet and it was gone within a week. But then we dealt with diaper yeast rash for a few months after that.

We introduced Sunshine to table foods around eight months of age. I would have delayed even longer, but she was ready! She followed her sisters' pattern of few solids until well over a year.

Sunshine is now twenty-two months old. She is nursing several times during the day and a couple of times at night. Since she is our last baby and I will not have a newborn after her, I may let her night-wean on her own.

Although Little Bit decreased her nursing, it was still getting too much for me to handle, so I have limited her to once in the morning and once before bed. It has been a couple of months since I have implemented that new rule, and she will still ask to nurse during the day. She is four years and five months old. She shows no interest in stopping nursing just yet. She told me recently she loves my milk because it is "cozy! And soooo healthy!"

I have learned a lot during this journey. I have learned patience. I have learned flexibility. I have learned that every child is different, even in the same family.

I have my favorite memories. Like when my older one would be nursing with the baby and reach out and hold or pat the baby's hand. She would smile around my nipple at her sister and I could just feel the love that flowed between them. I loved when my youngest was an infant and she would cry and my older girls would say "Momma, baby needs to nurse!" And I laugh when a toddler gets so excited to see a breast, that they clap and pounce on the nipple!

I have seen many benefits to breastfeeding. Comfort nursing a baby, or even an older toddler is a valid need. When my toddler would fall ill, nursing was the only thing they could eat and keep down. And it gave them the nutrition, fluids and antibodies they needed.

Throughout my journey my philosophy on babyhood and toddlerhood has grown and evolved. I have watched my girls strive for progress. I have watched them struggle to walk, finally accomplishing that after many falls. I have watched them go from needing me 24/7, to a slow shift in the other direction. And through all that I have seen that I do not need to push them to grow towards independence. I do not need to teach them how to learn and grow. I only need to support them as they do so, and to encourage them. I only need to give them an environment that helps them grow.

They will outgrow the need to nurse. Their need for that part of our relationship will slowly wane, until it is no longer a requirement. I see weaning as a developmental milestone, not a skill to be taught. When my girls are ready to move on from that, they will, with no need for me to decide for them.

In the meantime, I just enjoy the journey!

People say, 'You're still breastfeeding, that's so generous'. Generous,
no! It gives me boobs and takes my thighs away! It's sort of like
natural liposuction. I'd carry on breastfeeding for the rest of my life
if I could.

Helena Bonham-Carter

Breastfeeding is an unsentimental metaphor for how love works,
in a way. You don't decide how much and how deeply to love — you
respond to the beloved, and give with joy exactly as much as they
want.

Marni Jackson

Leeann's story

Erin was a honeymoon baby – born nine months and one week after our wedding. I had always thought that I would breastfeed, but I was not manic about it. I knew that it was the best thing for the child, according to all the research, so I felt a sense of responsibility as a parent-to-be to give it a go. I thought that it would be fine if I could breastfeed, but I wouldn't beat myself up if it didn't work out. My mum had given up breastfeeding me after a couple of days and there was no expectation from family about how I would feed my new baby. My mum was so excited to finally be getting a grandchild that how I fed it was the last thing on her mind! In early pregnancy my boobs really increased in size – it was a big early indicator of pregnancy for me. They've never gone back to their pre-pregnancy size.

When Erin was born she got stuck and after thirty-six hours of labour I had to have an extended episiotomy and forceps delivery. As a result of this, and the fact that Erin had a kidney condition that had been diagnosed via ultrasound earlier in the pregnancy, I had only a brief moment of skin-to-skin with her before they took her off to check her over, start her on antibiotics, and look at repairing me. They had to put a cannula in her hand as well. I was very relieved that she had been safely born, but I had been through the mill and eventually had to go to theatre for surgical repairs – under epidural. Up to that point I'd managed without the epidural! Jeb, my husband, was left alone in a blood-spattered room with baby Erin tucked inside his shirt. He had a good forty minutes to himself to get to know her and he looks back on that time he spent skin-to-skin with her very fondly now.

My memories of coming back from theatre are hazy but I can remember a midwife asking if I wanted to try to feed Erin. I was lying down and they put her against me, but I can't remember it being very successful, although they told me it was a 'good effort'. I was moved onto an observation ward because I was at higher risk due to blood loss and the extent of the repairs. Erin was with me all the time but I didn't have much help with the feeding. The first time I seriously tried to feed her was that evening, on the observation ward. Erin was screaming and I was beyond tired and getting very upset. I buzzed a nurse and just said "I can't do this". The nurse said "Shall we take her for a while so you can have a sleep?" I was so relieved that I fell asleep immediately and didn't wake until they brought Erin back several hours later. In retrospect I think they must have fed her formula while she was away from me, but they didn't say so and it didn't occur to me until much later.

It's in my nature to take my responsibilities seriously and just get on with what needs to be done. This means I don't always think to ask for help – I assume I am capable of most things. So I persevered with the breastfeeding without much support. I had felt very awkward while on a four-bed ward, with other people's visitors traipsing in and out, but once I was moved to a private room I relaxed a bit and stopped feeling as though Erin crying and me trying to feed her was disturbing everyone else. It was hard to get going with the breastfeeding in hospital. One health care assistant came in while I was trying to feed Erin and her comment was "Yes, well, you are rather large, aren't you?". My milk had come in by this point and my boobs were enormous. She showed me the 'rugby ball' hold (where the baby is propped up on pillows under your arm) and I found that much easier than the cross-cradle hold people had been recommending beforehand. She was also very 'hands-on' – something I wouldn't have thought I would be comfortable with – but it was fine under the circumstances.

Once we got home I didn't struggle too much with the feeding. I had cracked nipples but found the Lansinoh nipple cream that had been recommended by others to be fantastic – I can remember literally running upstairs to get some on so it would kill the pain. The sore nipples didn't last too long and I didn't worry too much about it because it seemed to be so common. I did have a few problems with engorgement, which I worried might turn into mastitis – my breasts would get hard and hot and I would have to express some milk off to soften the breast so that Erin could get latched on. I always had trouble remembering which side I was supposed to be feeding on next.

Within a couple of weeks of being home I felt we had the breastfeeding sorted out. I struggled then with the demands that breastfeeding made on me: it was difficult to adjust emotionally to Erin's constant need to be with me and me alone. After the difficult birth and ongoing recovery I was relieved that the feeding seemed to be going well. I was grateful for the NCT ante-natal classes I'd been to because they prepared me well for all these feelings and experiences – I knew what I was feeling was normal and that it would pass. I remember one day suddenly realising that I hadn't needed any nipple cream for several days.

I had always been determined that Erin would take a bottle and so, at around four weeks, I introduced a bottle of expressed milk. Later we tried her with formula to see if she would accept it. I couldn't help wanting to plan for disaster – what if something happened that meant I wasn't around to feed Erin? I had to know that she would be able to be fed by someone else. I was also pleased to be able to share the feeding with Jeb. I was always going to aim to feed Erin for six months – I had set that target for myself – but I never planned to do longer than that and so even from quite early on I was planning for the transition to bottles that would come later. I think your experience of breastfeeding really depends on your nature and I never saw myself as someone who would be in it for the long haul.

We drove to Northumbria from the Midlands when Erin was just a few weeks old and had to stop at a Little Chef when she needed a feed. It was the first time I had needed to feed her in public and I carefully chose a table in the corner but I still felt very uncomfortable. The rugby ball hold and the size of my boobs made it difficult to be discreet and I was always envious of other women who didn't seem to have the same problem. I never fed in front of any of my family – parents or siblings – preferring to go somewhere quiet and private. Fortunately Erin fed quickly so I didn't feel I was missing out on the conversation. I used to often take a bottle of expressed milk when I went out to avoid the whole issue of trying to feed and getting flustered. The only people I really fed in front of were Jeb, and my friends from the NCT group who were all in the same boat.

When Erin was two or three months old, Jeb and I went out for dinner for the first time, leaving Erin with my mum and a bottle of expressed milk. It hadn't occurred to me that not feeding for that three or four-hour period would mean that my boobs would leak, and I ended up sitting in the restaurant with my arms crossed over my chest to conceal the damp patches. I found that mortifying. I always got engorged when I was away from Erin for a while and it happened again after a black tie do that we went to in the December after Erin was born in August. I had planned to do the night feed when we got back but we were later arriving than I thought and by 1.30am when we finally got home I was in agony. I can remember hearing Erin stir a couple of minutes after we got home and I had never had her out of bed and on the boob so fast before – feeding her was such a relief.

Although I successfully established and continued breastfeeding, I never enjoyed feeding in public and never felt truly relaxed about it. I never worried about breastfeeding being the main way to bond with your baby – I'm sure I would have bonded just as well had we formula fed from the outset. I did feel some guilt at not having the preoccupation with breastfeeding that some mothers seem to have – I seem to have missed out on some of the 'warm and fuzzy' feelings that others report – although I always felt that it was nice enough. I can't imagine feeling the disappointment at not being able to feed, or the sadness when breastfeeding comes to an end, that I know others have experienced. For me breastfeeding was a fairly practical experience – I used to pride myself on getting out of bed, feeding Erin and getting us both back to bed within twenty minutes or so.

I knew that when Erin got to six months I was going to stop breastfeeding and I had a plan to do this. She had started solids by this point. On the day that she turned six months I did one last feed, in bed in the morning, and then simply stopped. She moved onto bottles with no fuss and I had no problems with engorgement because by then she was down to two feeds a day, in the morning and evening. She was a good eater and was only having three or four milk feeds in total.

Two things I found to be myths about breastfeeding – at least for me – were that it didn't seem to help with the weight loss, and I didn't drop a cup size when I stopped. Even now that Erin is four and going to school my boobs are still a size bigger than when I originally got pregnant!

In retrospect I think a lot of my feelings about breastfeeding stemmed from the fact that I couldn't manage to make the image of breastfeeding that I had in my head a reality – I was trying to live up to an ideal version of breastfeeding. I don't really know where I got this from, because before I had Erin I don't think I'd ever consciously observed anyone breastfeeding or even thought about it. I think women might find it easier to reconcile their feelings and the reality of breastfeeding if they saw more of it and got better support – at the moment each woman seems to be starting from scratch each time and our culture isn't very supportive. I think we have some romanticised notions of breast-feeding that aren't helpful when we're faced with the reality, and our society's suggestion that breastfeeding should be a private affair can make it difficult for women to ask for help. I learned through the experience of breastfeeding that my usual tactics of researching the theory and implementing it don't really cut it when it comes to something like breastfeeding – it's a skill that's learned best by getting hands-on help from others. When I look back I really wonder whether, if that health care assistant hadn't actually got her hands on my boobs and sorted us out with the rugby ball hold, I might have given up a lot sooner. It's hard to say for certain but that was definitely a turning point.

I strongly feel that when people make the decision to become parents they accept that their job is to do the best they can for their children. As such I find it very hard to understand those who won't even try to establish breastfeeding. No one ever pushed me to breastfeed – probably just as well, as I might have rebelled against it – but they didn't need to because rationally I knew it was the right thing to do, for me and for Erin. Despite my mixed feelings about some aspects of it, I feel very positive that it worked out for the six months I'd planned and confident that Erin had a great start in life.

Sonya's story

In my mid-twenties, long before I married and had my children, I had a breast cancer scare. I was very lucky to have only a short wait between my first consultation and biopsies and being given the diagnosis anyone in that position would want to have. They were benign tumours and needn't be removed unless I chose to. In those short few days, however, I went through the inevitable worries of what the future could hold for me. I remember, amongst those more obvious worries, that I was very concerned that should I need any surgery, it could affect my ability to breastfeed.

It is only now, some years on, that I realise that even back then, and without thinking, breastfeeding was a 'given' for me. I was emotionally signed up for it, before even needing to be intellectually informed and convinced. I knew that breastfeeding was going to be a pivotal part of what sort of mum I wanted to be. As having a family became a reality and I read about viewpoints ranging from feeding to 'the great nappy debate', I confirmed my feelings of breast being 'best for baby'. On every score (health, convenience, cost and environment), it won.

We were very excited going into my labour with Jessica and she was in a perfect position at the onset of labour. However, part way through she turned OP (back-to-back) and my labour slowed. After some time of incredible pain I agreed to a dose of pethidine, against my better judgment but begrudgingly accepted as I didn't want an epidural. After twenty-six hours of labour and a ventouse delivery, she was born healthy and we were all happy but exhausted. We had a little skin-to-skin contact and a small attempt at latching on, but I needed to sleep and did so for three hours whilst my husband cuddled and dozed with her.

All that day and night in hospital she was fussy about feeding and cried constantly, resisting me. I resorted to hand expressing a few drops of colostrum at a time and us giving it to her in a tiny cup in an attempt to quench her hunger enough to allow her to relax enough to feed. We struggled to get her latched on but we had lots of coaching from the hospital staff and she seemed to be making slow progress. The following morning, she gave a textbook demonstration, which gave us and our assigned midwife enough confidence to allow us home that day. That was the last textbook feed for some time.

Over the following few days we struggled to get her to latch on and stay there, regardless of what positions we tried. She remained fussy and sleepy yet disturbed and we continued to occasionally supplement with small amounts of expressed milk from a cup. This was not the bonding experience I had imagined it would be and I felt very disheartened, frustrated and like I was failing her. We were determined to carry on, however, and I retreated to my 'safe place' of methodical organisation. We noted down every attempt at a feed, how many seconds (yes, really!) she fed for and any expressed volumes we'd given her, her sleeps, her cries and her nappies. This was a double-edged sword as it gave me something to focus on but also highlighted in black and white how little she was feeding.

We were exhausted. Then my milk came in. I was hugely uncomfortable to add to it all.

The lowest point was later that week when we had an evening visit from friends to meet our new arrival. Soon after they arrived I went upstairs to feed Jessica. I was struggling to get her latched on and sat up there in the dark crying, trying in vain to get her to feed and therefore stop crying. Some time later my husband appeared and asked very quietly if I knew I'd been up there for two hours. I couldn't believe how long I'd been struggling and how I was beginning to lose perspective.

We had daily midwife/breastfeeding advisor visits for the first few days and that help was invaluable in that, along with the practical advice, it reassured me that I was not alone. They even phoned us to check how we were getting on. That help was above and beyond what I expected and I am very grateful for it. My husband was a rock too. He remained calm and collected, and ensured I had everything I needed 24/7 (even if it was just a hug) and reminded me of all the midwives' tips that I was too exhausted or too distressed to remember. He managed to find a great balance between hovering close enough while I fed to provide cushions/muslins and help with positioning and being a close part of it all, whilst managing to give me enough space to feel I wasn't being supervised.

We were determined to persevere. We knew it was right for Jessica and the pitbull in me doesn't like to be beaten.

Slowly, from around five or six days, the feeds began to be measured in minutes rather than seconds, my extreme discomfort reduced as my milk began to regulate, and the tiny expressed feeds were left behind. Jessica was able to get longer stretches of sleep as the 'too hungry to sleep, too tired to feed' cycle was broken down and she became increasingly relaxed.

After two weeks we resembled a fairly clued-up and well-practised breastfeeding family, and were discharged from midwife care with the proviso that we would continue to seek support if required. From that point we never looked back: she became a pleasure to feed with no colic and virtually no wind. She was a and a very clean and courteous baby to feed. I hit a stage when I got a very sore back, at around six weeks, but got through it as my muscles grew stronger and compensated. I learned quickly (with frequent nagging from my husband) that I should pay attention to a good feeding position or pay the price for a long time... I quickly became confident with feeding in public, learning how to express with a machine and even enjoying seeing my husband's bonding experience of feeding her expressed breast milk.

Despite a rocky start we had a really good feeding experience with Jessica. I had to learn to admit when I needed help and was grateful for the help and support we were given. I never questioned if we were doing the right thing, even when the going was very tough, and I'm so glad that we persevered.

*****

Given our difficult early days experience with Jessica, I entered my pregnancy with Oliver with a clear idea of what I did and didn't want out of my labour in order to do everything we could not have such a distressing breastfeeding experience again. I accepted that some of our previous experience was down to us both doing the learning curve but, justifiably or not, I attributed much of our experience to having had pethidine in labour.

I read extensively into the subject and concluded that much of Jessica's sleepiness and fussiness was likely to be caused by pethidine and, of course, the long labour. I contacted my labour ward and asked if they would administer an alternative, lower half-life, opiate-based drug and they said "no". This (and the fact that I was told I was having a big baby and might need to be induced, making it highly likely that I would need some very purposeful pain relief planned!) gave me a mission. So I made appointments to speak to the consultant anaesthesiologists at three other major hospitals in the region, choosing not to rely solely on the internet for my information. We then had a very inspiring meeting with the CA at my hospital (once I had convinced them that I had done my research, knew enough to not be wasting their time and, crucially, was not going to let it drop). During a long meeting, she agreed to offer me an alternative drug, but very supportively concluded that I should strongly consider a water birth.

To cut a long story short (very short), I went into labour naturally and, after only one hour and forty-five minutes, Oliver was born in a blissful, drug-free, water birth. We hadn't even got the overnight bag out of the car... It was one of the most magical experiences of my life.

Within four hours of birth he was on his fourth feed, he didn't cry and he slept sweetly for the rest of the day. Through the following days he quickly got into a routine and fed well at almost every feed. When my milk came in it was even more intense than before. My boobs were as hard as rock, you could almost hear them go "dink" when you tapped them. You could certainly feel the heat radiating from them from some inches away and lying on my side was impossible. Oliver fed so well though that it took only a few days to regulate, for which I am thankful, as lifting and cuddling two-year-old Jessica was excruciating. For the first month he was textbook, if a little pukey, compared to Jessica.

At four weeks he was developing a behaviour that looked like the onset of colic and had become very pukey (both of us needing two or three changes of clothes every day, muslins stashed in every nook and cranny of the house and a small reluctance on my part to feed in public). We began to look at everything from my diet to our routine and winding techniques but couldn't get to the bottom of it. At this point he was crying a lot during the evenings and difficult to settle to sleep after night-time feeds and we were beginning to feel worried about how long it would last and how it was to affect our sanity.

Oliver got himself through the wind/colic by ten weeks, as nothing we did changed anything. At nearly four months old he remains a pukey baby, though it is much less intense. We still have one day in five where I am sponging down the sofa and mopping the floor of milk though!

I am really enjoying feeding again and we are so pleased with how well we have got up and running, being so comfortable and relaxed with feeding so early. We are particularly pleased with Oliver's weight gain, being mostly an average of one once per day. We must be doing something right!

*****

Weaning

I went on to feed Jessica for over a year. I knew I would aim for a minimum of six months, and as six months came and went we just carried on. From her third month my husband enjoyed giving her bottles of expressed milk once or sometimes twice a week at her evening feed and, although a little odd for me at first, it became fun to enjoy a glass of wine whilst he did it! She was weaned at six months, but her milk feeds continued to come from me. At nine months I returned to work and, with regret, we introduced formula for her nursery feeds (the thought of expressing that volume whilst back to nearly full-time work was too much for me). I continued to give her all her feeds outside of nursery until she weaned herself off at thirteen months. She had become increasingly fussy and uninterested from about eleven months and, although it tugged at my heartstrings, I could see the end of our feeding relationship looming. It was the right time to stop, though. She was ready and eventually I realised that I was too.

We intend for me to breastfeed Oliver for at least twelve months, as we did Jessica. However, already I can tell he is a hungrier, heavier and more fidgety baby, so we'll see how easy it is to stay the distance this time or if he decides to self-wean earlier than Jessica did.

Breastfeeding after-sales

Jessica was 8lb when she was born and maintained a steady weight gain. I took her to Baby Clinic regularly to get her weighed. After a few weeks it seemed that she was reaching a plateau and not gaining weight according to the centile graph in her red book. My experience with health visitors was very mixed but, on the whole, disappointing. They felt that she should be putting on weight quicker. I'd heard that the graph in use at the time was based on bottle-fed babies, who gain weight quicker than exclusively breastfed babies. I therefore asked if perhaps the graph was not appropriate for Jessica and that her weight gain was not as slow as the graph made out. I asked for a graph for breast-fed babies, but it was not forthcoming. The health visitors were puzzled and somewhat indignant.

It was at that point that I realised that the after-sales service on breastfeeding was not as good as the pre-sales! I sought out the appropriate graph myself and charted Jessica's weight against both graphs at every weigh-in. Every time they raised an eyebrow about her weight gain, I referred them to the breast-fed baby chart and they begrudgingly (because it didn't fit their 'norm') agreed that her weight gain was sufficient. She is now two and following a healthy centile.

Friends' preconceptions

Some of my friends, who had children of similar ages, had feeding problems that caused them to decide to quit breastfeeding. I'm sure they felt uncomfortable discussing this due to their feelings of guilt, as my early experience had been similar yet I had persevered. I felt this drove a divide between us as they had preconceptions around whether I would judge them over their decision. I tried not to judge and tried to offer advice where I felt it would be welcome and also went by the mantra that 'a stressed out mum makes a stressed out baby'. I hope this helped at the time but I still get the odd comment that leads me to believe that they cannot truly discuss the issue with me.

Drinking and feeding

I am a notable lover of a tipple or two. I was very upset one day, whilst pregnant with Jessica, when a friend remarked seriously that I wouldn't feed for long as I wouldn't be able to resist red wine. This really upset me and made me determined to prove him wrong, and I did. However, I also learned that being a breastfeeding mum does not mean complete abstinence – the key is in the timing! In my opinion it is fine to have a beer or glass of wine just after a feed, if you know baby will not be feeding again in a while!*

Health benefits

One of the main arguments for breastfeeding is that babies benefit from better health (fewer colds, ear infections, tummy bugs etc). I can say that Jessica only had one cold and one twenty-four-hour bug, no ear infections and no other illnesses of any sort for twelve months, including her first three months at nursery, when they are subjected to all sorts of germs. She didn't have paracetamol until she was nine months and has never needed any other medication. We are not draconian enough to deny her any medication if she needs it, nor are we soft enough to hide her away from any possible contact with bugs and sniffles. The simple fact is she is not an ill child and Oliver seems to be following in her footsteps. Read into that what you wish!

We feel proud that we are giving our children the best start in life that we can and are enjoying the closeness, health and convenience that breastfeeding provides.

With his small head pillowed against your breast and your milk warming his insides, your baby knows a special closeness to you. He is gaining a firm foundation in an important area of life — he is learning about love.

La Leche League pamphlet, c.1956

In breastfeeding, the infant is cradled in the mother's arms. Pleasure in sucking, the satisfaction of hunger, intimacy with the mother's body, are united with his recognition of her face.

Selma Fraiberg

Ali's story

The woman writing this story was never going to have children! Something sometime when I was a girl scared me rigid about the whole pregnancy thing and as I was never that keen on children (even when I was one) there seemed no reason to get over my phobia. Yet here in 2011 I have two daughters aged three and eleven months and both are still breastfed. Having been the least maternal person I knew I am now known to my new friends and colleagues as 'the earth mother'!

Breastfeeding has been a significant part of my transformation yet I have approached it in the same way I do most things in my life, with lots of lists, reading up and if absolutely necessary asking for help! I remember being asked at my hospital booking appointment how I was expecting to feed my baby and asking the midwife back "well I don't know much about it, could you tell me the benefits?" She shocked me as she reeled off loads of health benefits for mothers that I had never heard of and no "breast is best" cliché at all. If I am honest though the thing that swung it for me was that it is natural and free. Why would I want to give myself hassle and expense to expose my child to the risks of what is, by definition, a replacement?

Before my daughter (DD) was born, I read and read about how to feed, how to overcome problems and even how to handle big boobs, as my pair, even before breastfeeding, would give some of the "enhanced" women on *Eurotrash* a run for their money. I had DD in an induced hospital birth that was not really how I planned it, but the one thing I achieved was immediate skin-to-skin. She was birthed, brought up on to my chest and I fed her almost immediately as I held her next to my heart to start our breastfeeding relationship.

Over the next few days she fed alright, but I really struggled to know how to hold her and was scared of smothering her. I looked at all the pictures and videos online I could but somehow I could not replicate any of the positions. I just felt I needed an extra pair of hands. Luckily a home visit midwife pointed out that babies "flare" their nostrils and that is how they are built, so I got over that initial worry and relaxed.

When she got to three weeks old I just felt I was cracking things. I could feed out and about as long as I had a cardigan to roll up as a makeshift pillow to prop her on, I felt an old hand at the other baby stuff like nappies and I was mastering one-handed eating, when she suddenly went 'bonkers'. Having just begun to feel 'in tune' with my daughter I suddenly could not do anything right. All my notes and lists showed me I was not doing anything different yet she was not happy! This was growth spurt number one. Once I gave in, chucked my lists away, trusted her and my instinct and unclipped the nursing bra, even if I had only stopped feeding her five minutes earlier, then bingo she was happy. And so was I! Phew! I had learnt my first real lesson as a mother: as much as I wanted me and my spreadsheets to be in control, DD was really in the driving seat.

My advance reading on a breastfeeding support forum did help though, as I became prepared for the natural progressions of feeding. I was aware that I would have times when I doubted my supply but I knew to just feed and feed and I got through those high-demand periods. When DD would feed for over an hour at a time, coming off after twenty minutes or so to just go back on for another course a few minutes later, I realised this was normal for her. I also, a few months down the line, managed to resist the temptations of early introduction of solids and successfully follow a baby-led approach from when she reached twenty-five weeks.

In amongst the experiences of my new online friends I came across the concept of milk banking. I already had a breast pump as we were giving a bottle of expressed milk a couple of times a week at bedtime, so it seemed quite reasonable to me to just pump more and send it to the 'poorly' babies. I started when DD was about seven weeks old and would pump every morning, hopefully before she woke up, putting a bottle in the freezer. I was lucky that she slept well, so more often than not by getting up before 7am I would manage to pump before she demanded her morning fill. Every few weeks a volunteer would bring over some new bottles to fill and take away my contribution to the Wirral Mothers' Milk bank. I continued right up to DD's first birthday, though by this time, having gone back to work, I was finding it harder to fill my bottles and pump enough for my daughter to have whilst away from me. I was so proud of myself though, especially as they sent me a certificate saying I had donated nearly thirty-two litres!

As the months went on my mummy friends gradually introduced more and more replacements to breast milk and stopped feeding. Unusually three of my real-life friends continued past their child's first birthday, but I saw no reason to stop. My daughter just seemed so happy with the situation of typically three or four feeds a day when she was with me and I was happy to continue. We did have a very awkward time when she was fifteen or sixteen months and sprouting her first teeth. It seemed to change her latch so on one side it really hurt!

My periods had come back when DD was about nine months old, so when my husband joked that he would get me pregnant so that I had to drive on New Year's Eve, it was a possibility. It worked!

This time at my booking-in appointment when they asked about breastfeeding I was able to say I was still feeding DD and got 'experienced mother' written in the breastfeeding section of my notes. There were a few weeks of the pregnancy when feeding DD made me feel just yucky, but I had no option but to close my eyes and continue as she was becoming more verbal by the day and she clearly wanted mummy milk. I got the benefits though as once I reduced my hours towards the end of my pregnancy and then started my maternity leave my now two-year-old needed an afternoon nap but would not really take one. Her mummy desperately needed one, so I tended to feed her lying on the floor in the living room and we would both drift off to the sounds of CBeebies!

The evening I was in labour with E I even fed DD to sleep. I loved the fact I had nurtured her that far and that although she was going to have to share from then on, she could have one more evening of me to herself. I will admit to closing my eyes through a few contractions though!

E was born the next morning in a pool in our conservatory whilst DD slept upstairs. Within a minute or so of coming up into the air E was attached... like a cyclone vacuum cleaner! She stayed attached for the next hour and was feeding so well you could even hear her swallowing! I suppose that having continued to feed DD my colostrum was in a greater volume than the usual few drops of nectar.

E did give me a few minutes peace through that first day, but I knew from then that she was a different kettle of fish to her sister. No mammoth feeding sessions: she was a little but very, very often girl. She hardly slept, even during the day, so there was no 'get her off to sleep and rush around like a mad woman to get stuff done' lark like when I had DD. For starters I had DD around and two-year-olds take a lot of placating, but also E would basically feed wherever I was and whatever I was doing. I fed her round the supermarket (when she was one-day-old and two-days-old and many times since, including today), I have fed her whilst walking round railway museums, cathedrals, safari parks and on the beach.

We went camping when E was nearly six weeks old and with breastfeeding and using a sling it was really easy! We even use cloth nappies when camping, which some people reckon is a bit weird, but it is really so easy. As long as E had me and my boobies she was happy! Well, happy-ish! I suspect she had mild reflux as she was quite sicky and there were times when I knew she was feeding not because of hunger but because it soothed her. Many mums I know would have rushed to 'diagnose' and medicate and probably blame themselves, but I knew it was just one of those things and E was just a noisier and less straightforward to please girl than her big sister.

On returning from camping I started pumping for the milk bank as I had done with DD, but this time it was different. For starters it is harder to get up between 6 and 7am to pump when you have been up five, six or seven times in the night feeding and generally being a mum! Also my boobs and their production are just different. In the early days they were on mega drive! I suppose from feeding DD they were well up to speed and well up to the task of filling the odd 4oz bottle or two as well. More recently I have found it a real struggle to face pumping when completely knackered and seemingly drunk dry. E has only recently started sleeping better at night, and waking means mummy milk is required. At about seven months she improved a little so I was up to her maybe four or five times, and more recently it is usually two or maybe three times. I know some people would 'blame' breast feeding for this, but I know it is just how some babies are and at least I have the easy soporific elixir on tap and thank goodness I am not reliant on having to measure and sterilise and warm and cool.

Even though it is some people's magic, a bottle has not helped. She refused all alternative feeding methods up to about five months, when we tried the basic bottle that came with my pump. From then on my husband was able to take a different part of bedtime in that he could do E a couple or three times a week whilst I sorted DD. It has given me the option to go out on a few occasions too, though mainly for the early part of the evening, and I have had to continue to feed her through the night.

Introducing solids has not helped either. She feeds a little less during the day, as there is only so much time between fistfuls of pasta, peaches and strawberries, but in spite of being a very enthusiastic baby-led weaner from the day she was six months old she has continued to need her mummy milk for both nutrition and comfort.

I am lucky that my husband supports my choice to breastfeed and do baby-led weaning. I will acknowledge though that although my reasons are down to sound research and consideration of the risks of 'the other way', he probably likes breastfeeding and baby-led weaning because it gives him an easy life! He can get on with his tea whilst I feed (eating one-handed myself) and these days everyone eats the same meal at the same time.

So I come to my second born nearing her first birthday and my first born still enjoying her mummy milk, albeit just a couple of times a week. I have no idea when DD will self-wean, but pregnancy didn't do it… wonder if I should try that again?

I know I will have at least a few more months ahead where I can't plan an outfit for a special occasion that does not include access arrangements for E and just at the time when my friends also on their second babies are moving back into lovely uplifting bras I find I can justify a new nursing bra to replace the greying one that is not fit to be seen as it will get plenty of wear.

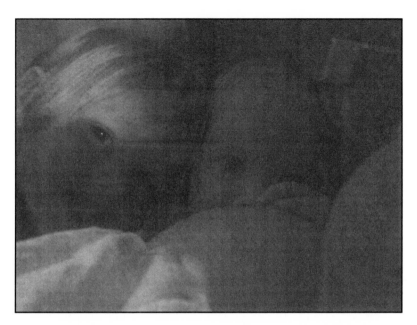

I am back at work again and pumping for E though she has not taken any whilst at nursery as there are just too many things to eat and play with. Mind you, as soon as she catches sight of me she flings her head to one side and almost climbs inside my top! She is still keen!

Soon the poorly babies will not want my pumped magic juice either (you have to stop at twelve months for my milk bank) but I will continue feeding my walking talking babies until they choose to stop.

I'm like an alcoholic. It's like, I don't care if I cry, I don't care if I'm fat, I'm just gonna do it for one more week, one more month, and then, when I see how much good it is doing her, I can't stop. It's a very powerful thing you know.

Salma Hayek

I lost most of my weight from breastfeeding and I encourage women to do it; it's just so good for the baby and good for yourself.

Beyoncé

How to get help

In the first instance speak to your midwife or health visitor. They may be able to put you in touch with an infant feeding advisor or breastfeeding coordinator based at your local hospital, particularly if it is baby-friendly.

There may be an active peer support network in your area (eg Breast Buddies, Little Angels etc). You can find this out via midwives/health visitors, Children's Centres, or by searching online. Other local mothers can be an invaluable source of support.

To find your nearest IBCLC (International Board Certified Lactation Consultant) visit the LCGB (Lactation Consultants Great Britain) page at www.lcgb.org

The major breastfeeding charities run helplines that you can call for information and support. They are staffed by experienced volunteers who have had training in supporting breastfeeding.

LA LECHE LEAGUE

www.laleche.org.uk
Helpline: 0845 120 2918

ASSOCIATION OF BREASTFEEDING MOTHERS (ABM)

www.abm.me.uk
Helpline: call 08444 122 949 to speak to a fully trained breastfeeding counsellor (9.30am-10.30pm)

NCT

www.nct.org.uk
Breastfeeding helpline: 0300 330 0771 (seven days a week, 8am-10pm)

THE BREASTFEEDING NETWORK

www.breastfeedingnetwork.org.uk
Helpline: 0300 100 0210 (9.30am-9.30pm every day)
Drugs in Breastmilk helpline **0844 412 4665 (see notes on the website)**

GOVERNMENT HELPLINE

Manned by The Breastfeeding Network and Association of Breastfeeding Mothers: 0300 100 0212

Further reading

Dr Jack Newman, *The Ultimate Breastfeeding Book of Answers*, Three Rivers Press, New York, 2000

Gabrielle Palmer, *The Politics of Breastfeeding*, Pinter and Martin, 2009

La Leche League International, *The Womanly Art of Breastfeeding*, Pinter and Martin, 2010

Kate Evans, *Food of Love*, Myriad Editions, 2008

Ina May Gaskin, *Ina May's Guide to Breastfeeding*, Pinter and Martin, 2009

Gill Rapley and Tracey Murkett, *Baby-Led Weaning – Teaching Your Baby To Love Good Food*, Vermilion, London, 2008

Alison Blenkinsop, *Fit to Bust: A Comic Treasure Chest*, Lonely Scribe, 2011

Ann Sinnot, *Breastfeeding Older Children*, Free Association Books, 2009

Valerie Finigan, *Saggy Boobs and other Breastfeeding Myths*, Pinter and Martin, 2009

Elizabeth Pantley, *The No Cry Sleep Solution – Gentle Ways to Help Your Baby Sleep Through The Night*, McGraw Hill, 2002.

I have given suck, and know
How tender 'tis to love the babe that milks me

Shakespeare, Macbeth, *Act II, Scene I*

He saw a girl working about the stove, saw that she carried a baby
on her crooked arm, and that the baby was nursing, its head up
under the girl's shirtwaist. And the girl moved about, poking the
fire, shifting the rusty stove lids to make a better draft, opening the
oven door; and all the time the baby sucked, and the mother shifted
it deftly from arm to arm. The baby didn't interfere with her work or
with the quick gracefulness of her movements.

John Steinbeck, The Grapes of Wrath, *Chapter 21*

The mothers shall give suck to their offsprings, for two complete years.

Quran Surah II (Baqarah) Verse 233

Online resources

Breastfeeding support

www.kellymom.com
Evidence-based information written by an IBCLC.

www.howbreastfeedingworks.com
Mythbusting, informative website

www.mumsnet.com
Mumsnet – see the breast and bottle feeding forum for help with all feeding questions.

www.analyticalarmadillo.co.uk
Very informative blog written by breastfeeding counsellor.

www.nct.org.uk/parenting/feeding-0
NCT breastfeeding pages

Breastfeeding – wider issues

www.who.int/topics/breastfeeding/en/
World Health Organisation pages on breastfeeding.

www.unicef.org.uk/BabyFriendly/
Unicef Baby Friendly initiative.

www.babymilkaction.org
Baby Milk Action: protecting breastfeeding, protecting babies fed on formula.

Also available from Lonely Scribe

HOME BIRTHS
stories to inspire and inform

A moving collection of real life stories celebrating the joy and wonder of birth at home. This collection of first-hand recollections by mothers and their partners gives an insight into the modern experience of home birth, from the first decision to the final push.

ISBN 978-1-905179-02-2 •
£13.99/$24.99

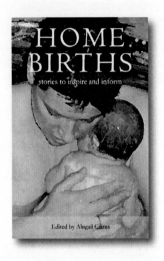

FIT TO BUST
a comic treasure chest

Fit to Bust is a treasury of bits and boobs to celebrate motherhood and breastfeeding. Proceeds from its sale will support Baby Milk Action in its endeavour to protect breastfeeding, and protect all babies, however they are fed.

'It's exactly what it says on the tin. A comic treasure chest, and very funny. Bravo.'

ISBN 978-1-905179-02-2 •
£13.99/$24.99

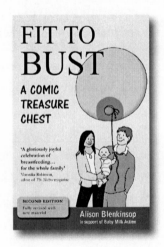

ORDER FORM

Order

☐ Please send me _____ copies of *Home Births* at a cost of £13.99 each

☐ Please send me _____ copies of *Fit to Bust* at a cost of £12.99 each

☐ Please send me _____ copies of *Breastfeeding* at a cost of £13.99 each

Payment

☐ I enclose a cheque for _____

Delivery is free within the UK. Contact us to find out about international delivery charges.

Delivery and contact details

Name: _____

Address: _____

_____

_____

Telephone: _____

Email: _____

Please make cheques payable to **Lonely Scribe**, and return to:
Welwyn, Bermuda Avenue, Little Eaton, Derbyshire DE21 5DG

To check receipt of your order form or find out about a delivery date
call **01453 488500** or email **contact@lonelyscribe.co.uk**

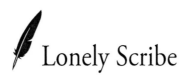

Lonely Scribe

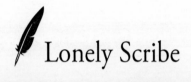 Lonely Scribe

ORDER FORM

Order

☐ Please send me _____ copies of *Home Births* at a cost of £13.99 each

☐ Please send me _____ copies of *Fit to Bust* at a cost of £12.99 each

☐ Please send me _____ copies of *Breastfeeding* at a cost of £13.99 each

Payment

☐ I enclose a cheque for _____

Delivery is free within the UK. Contact us to find out about international delivery charges.

Delivery and contact details

Name: _____

Address: _____

_____

_____

Telephone: _____

Email: _____

Please make cheques payable to **Lonely Scribe**, and return to:
Welwyn, Bermuda Avenue, Little Eaton, Derbyshire DE21 5DG

To check receipt of your order form or find out about a delivery date
call **01453 488500** or email **contact@lonelyscribe.co.uk**

Lightning Source UK Ltd.
Milton Keynes UK
UKOW050816110612

194208UK00001B/4/P